Comprehensive review for the

RADIOLOGIC TECHNOLOGIST

Mosby's comprehensive review series

Other books available

Dolan: *Comprehensive Review for* MEDICAL TECHNOLOGISTS
Goodman & Schoedinger: *Questions and Answers in* ORTHOPAEDICS, 2nd ed.
Gutch & Stoner: *Review of* HEMODIALYSIS FOR NURSES AND DIALYSIS PERSONNEL
Hartstein: *Questions and Answers on* CONTACT LENS PRACTICE
Hartstein: *Review of* REFRACTION
Hine: *Review of* DENTISTRY, *Questions and Answers*, 5th ed.
Hurtt, Rasicovici & Windsor: *Comprehensive Review of* ORTHOPTICS AND OCULAR MOTILITY
Lawton & Foy: *Comprehensive Review for the* MEDICAL ASSISTANT
Meyer & Steinberg: *Review of* LABORATORY MEDICINE
Mosby's *Comprehensive Review of* NURSING, 7th ed.
Mosby's *Review of* PRACTICAL NURSING, 4th ed.
Peterson: *Comprehensive Review for* DENTAL HYGIENISTS, 2nd ed.
Peterson & Winnett: *Review and Test Manual for* DENTAL ASSISTANTS

Books to be published

Bergersen: *Comprehensive Review of* PHARMACOLOGY IN NURSING
Burnett & Schuster: *Review of* PATHOGENIC MICROBIOLOGY
Howard: *Review of* CLINICAL OPERATIVE DENTISTRY
Reinecke, Stein & Slatt: *Introductory Manual of the* OPHTHALMIC ASSISTANT
Williams: *Review of* NUTRITION AND DIET THERAPY

Comprehensive review for the
RADIOLOGIC TECHNOLOGIST

Matthew Stevens, R.T.

Director, Radiologic Technology, Northeastern University, Boston, Massachusetts

Robert I. Phillips, R.T., FASRT

Director of Radiologic Services, The Methodist Hospital, Houston, Texas

Second edition

With 19 illustrations

The C. V. Mosby Company
Saint Louis   1972

PREFACE

This book has been prepared in the hope that it will aid the student technologist and contribute to technology in general. We believe it is a book that the technologist may use to gain a knowledge of his chosen vocation and for purposes of passing the National Registry Examination. We have tried to cover the fundamentals of radiologic technology that are essential to advancement or for performance of daily duties.

It is our hope that this book will be used in conjunction with the numerous texts already available to the student and technologist. It is our aim that after the technologist uses the available books and assimilates the material, this book will then become more important as a reference. We have assembled the subject matter in question and answer form so that important facts and techniques will be readily accessible. But to take advantage of our format, the student must have learned the fundamentals previously.

This second edition has been expanded and updated, particularly in those sections dealing with medical and radiologic terminology, anatomy and physiology, medical-surgical diseases, radiation protection and therapy, and radioactive isotopes. We hope these additions will serve to acquaint the student with the latest information available in his field and will, especially with the inclusion of a second simulated registry examination, serve as a more thorough review text.

During the past few years technology has made progress that has astounded the medical profession. This progress is but a prelude of the things to come. If the technologist is to grow with the profession, he must equip himself to meet the demands that are being made and those that will be made in the future. We feel that this preparation can best be accomplished by adequate educational and practical experience. These two aspects cannot be separated because each has its own effect upon the formation of a well-trained technologist.

There are still areas of disagreement within the medical profession regarding the amount of education required for the technologist. Those opposed to increased education are, hopefully, in the minority; the other faction feels that through education the technologist will be better able to assume the responsibilities thrust upon him, and therefore the entire profession will prosper and patient care will improve.

We must never be satisfied with our level of education. We must continue to learn and progress; otherwise, we will stagnate and fall by the way. It is sincerely hoped that this book will take its place with other technology books and assist in continued educational advancement.

For permission to reproduce copyrighted material special acknowledgement is given to GAF Corporation for use of their questions and answers in the publication *Automatic Processing of X-ray Film;* Joseph Selman, M.D., and Charles C Thomas, Publisher, for the use of diagrams of Transformer Types; General Electric Company, X-ray Department, for reproductions of diagrams, drawings, and questions from that company's technical service publications; and Leibel Flarsheim Company for reproduction of their material on grids.

To the many technologists and student technologists who have reviewed and criticized the material and made valuable suggestions, we extend our thanks.

To our respective institutions, Northeastern University and The Methodist Hospital, we are appreciative of the time allowed to work on the projects and the encouragement given by them. A special word of thanks is given to Dr. Laurence L. Robbins, Radiologist-in-Chief, Massachusetts General Hospital, for his efforts in spurring us on.

MATTHEW STEVENS
ROBERT I. PHILLIPS

CONTENTS

Appendix

Comprehensive review for the

RADIOLOGIC TECHNOLOGIST

INTRODUCTION

Technologists have every reason to be proud of the profession they have selected and, because it has been their choice, to strive constantly to ensure its remaining on the high professional level it enjoys today. Only by the constant efforts of those within the profession can it continue to grow and prosper.

Since the discovery of x-rays by Professor Roentgen about seventy-five years ago, their importance to the health profession has steadily progressed until today x-rays are highly respected and widely used. In the beginning they were the cause of many cartoons and jokes claiming they would never be of any use. This has been proved false since many new procedures and techniques are directly attributed to the use of x-rays. They have allowed for and assisted in gaining knowledge of anatomy and physiology that might otherwise have been overlooked or would have required a greater amount of time and study.

The general public and some within the medical field have little knowledge about the properties and uses of x-radiation. Too often published articles to which the public has access are couched in terms that create doubt and fear rather than assurance of the beneficial uses for which x-rays are applied. The impression received by the reader is one of danger. While it is true that a certain danger is present, properly administered radiation can assist in obtaining radiographs that, when interpreted, can be a valuable tool in the diagnosis and prognosis of the patient. It is the responsibility of those in the profession to educate the public and other related medical areas to the nature of the radiologic profession.

The technologist should avail himself of every opportunity to explain to patients and other groups of interested persons the nature of x-rays and the many benefits humanity has received from them. The technologist has a responsible position and one that should never be taken lightly. His colleagues who are in related medical areas such as nursing, laboratories, dentistry, dietetics, and medicine should be encouraged to discuss one another's duties and responsibilities. Technologists should belong to their professional organizations and attend lectures, seminars, and classes to obtain current information, which should also be beneficial for improving qualifications for advancement. This growth and advancement will occur within the individual as well as professionally.

Again we would like to point out that it is the responsibility of every technologist to educate the other related medical areas, patients, and the public about his duties and the nature of radiation. The successful

1

technologist has pride in his skill, profession, and achievements, as well as in the position that he enjoys in the overall health team. The technologist should be proud of his position on the team and should strive constantly to continue the excellent tradition and heritage of which he is an integral part.

1 THE AMERICAN REGISTRY OF RADIOLOGIC TECHNOLOGISTS

The American Registry of Radiologic Technologists was first organized in 1922 under the joint sponsorship of the Radiological Society of North America, the American Roentgen Ray Society, the Canadian Association of Radiologists, and the American Society of X-ray Technicians.

Members of these organizations recognized the need for a standard of training to develop technicians capable of producing better technical work and to establish a better rapport between the radiologist and the technologist.

In 1936 the Registry was incorporated as the American Registry of X-ray Technicians. In 1944 the Radiological Society of North America relinquished its sponsorship in favor of the American College of Radiology; also in 1944 the American Medical Association's Council on Education assumed the functions of inspection, approval, and listing of qualified schools of x-ray technology. The Advisory Committee of the American College of Radiology and the Education Committee of the American Society of Radiologic Technologists created a basic curriculum and teacher's syllabus as another step in standardizing training in approved schools of x-ray technology.

The primary function and purpose of the Registry is to prepare and administer examinations for persons having graduated from approved training schools. Certification by the Registry means that the person has met all the basic requirements, is of good moral character, and is therefore eligible to practice the art and science of radiologic technology.

During the early days of radiology and technology, training was somewhat haphazard, and almost anyone with a moderate amount of intelligence could be taught to operate the equipment. The rapid advances achieved by the profession soon made this method of training obsolete, and those within the profession with enough initiative and foresight recognized the need for having a standard training program. Over the years basic training standards have been advanced and are still being elevated. Radiologists and technologists must undergo rigid training for many years. Now two-year training-approved schools, which must supply specific basic knowledge in certain subject areas, are available. Any school wishing to train technologists must meet certain requirements to be eligible, and graduates of these schools must apply to the Registry for certification. The Registry will evaluate the application, and, if the criteria have been met, then the registry will notify the applicant of the time and place at which the examination will be given. Initially, examinations were given to applicants at almost any time since the examination was forwarded to a radiologist who would administer it to the technologist in his presence. This system became outdated, and today examinations are offered twice a year, the first weekends of May and November. All applicants, graduates of approved schools, are assigned specific dates on which to take the examinations.

Perhaps we should elaborate more on the specifics regarding an approved school. An approved school is one that has as its director a board-certified radiologist who makes application to the Council of Medical Education of the American Medical Association for approval. The hospital (since most schools are hospital based) must follow the teacher's syllabus for course content and must perform a specific number of examinations of all types to be eligible for approval. If all criteria are met, then an inspection team composed of one radiologist and one technologist will visit the school for an on-the-site inspection. They will interview the director, chief technologist, technologist, and students and review records and reports of the students and the department. The inspecting team will submit individual reports to the Joint Review Committee. This Joint Review Committee (cosponsored by the American College of Radiology and the American Society of Radiologic Technologists) will review the inspection reports and make recommendations to the Council on Medical Education of the American Medical Association. If all is in order, approval is given to the school by the Council. If not, deficencies are pointed out and time to repair or correct them is given. At the end of the allotted time the school is again visited and specific deficiencies noted previously are checked for correction. If they are found to be corrected, then approval is given.

Because of the rapid growth during the last few years, colleges and universities are actively involved in preparing technologists. Students are attending classes at the educational institution for theory and some practice. Although this somewhat relieves the burden of lecturing on the hospitals, they are still required to supply a minimum amount of lecture hours and the practicum. These relationships are working well and improving constantly. After the student completes these approved programs, the Registry will evaluate the applications and supply the examinations for certification. Successfully passing the examination entitles the person to enter the profession as a technologist. He must agree to work only under the supervision of a physician who is acceptable to the Board of Trustees and under no circumstances to give written or oral diagnosis.

In radiology, as in most areas of medicine, specialization has come into being. Today the field includes medical radiologic technology, nuclear medicine technology, and radiation therapy technology. The Registry must also examine and certify as proficient persons in these areas. They also have basic minimum requirements to meet and uphold. The Registry must constantly be alert to the elevation of the entire profession and must increase the requirements for attaining registration consistent with the professional growth and improvement of service to patients.

The Board of Trustees has the right to refuse renewal or certification of any person accused or found guilty of violation of the code of ethics. Every person has the right of appearing before the board in person or submitting a written affidavit as to why certification should not be withheld. Any person against whom a complaint has been filed will be notified at least thirty days in advance about the nature of the complaint and the meeting date on which the complaint will be heard.

Any certificate that has been revoked

may be reissued after compliance with the requirements of the Board of Trustees.

Every student or graduate should apply for certification and after receiving it should join the American Society of Radiologic Technologists and actively participate in its operation. This is the method by which technology will continue to meet and exceed the standards of performance required of it. It is recognized that some persons presently are not in agreement with established policies and procedures; this is healthy as long as they exercise their rights and objections in an orderly, judicial, democratic way and strive for improvement and elevation of their profession.

Both the Registry and the Society are comprised of persons elected or appointed to office. They wish to serve the needs of the profession and its members to the best of their abilities. If you do not agree with present procedures, then feel free to criticize, but be sure that your comments are constructive and not destructive. Constructive criticism is welcomed and invited.

Technologists should support the Registry and Societies and work actively to advance them.

2 HOW TO PREPARE FOR THE NATIONAL REGISTRY EXAMINATION

Preparing for and taking the National Registry Examination may well be the mountaintop experience in students' lives. Certainly, they have taken many examinations in high school and postgraduate education. However, this is the big one, and school did not prepare them to master the ability of examination taking.

Examinations are often called "seances," the recalling of the departed. Students complain that the instructor gives the examination to be relieved of teaching that session. It has been said that an examination is a two-way street. It shows what the teacher has taught and what the student has learned. All students have longed for the day when something will replace the examination in testing ability and recall. Today a movement has been initiated to eliminate the marking system in education, but for now examinations are here to stay.

When talking to people about examination taking, students are likely to say that everything they knew left when the examination took place. What they are saying is that their minds went blank. Others have been known to become violently ill, even to the point of vomiting. If all the obvious complaints are analyzed, fear is found to be the underlying motive. Students fear not knowing the answers and thus failing the examination.

It was perhaps Bette Davis who once said that all good actors and actresses have butterflies in their stomachs as they await their cue.

The speaker's fear is manifest in many ways, even when he has carefully prepared and written his speeches. Few persons are completely confident when called upon to say a few words before a large room filled with people. A well-known technologist once said, "Remember that you know more about the subject than they do." This may not always be true, and if the speaker assumes this attitude, the audience is likely to resent it.

In public speaking courses it is maintained that the speaker should reach his audience, become a part of it. A great many speakers attempt to reach the audience by telling humorous stories. Some express how happy they are that they were invited to be present and to appear on the program. Some speakers, confident that no one knows the subject as well as themselves, just begin with the subject matter. This overcoming of fear changes the attitude of the speaker toward his audience. If we are truly realistic, no one speaker can

6

know more about his subject than every-one in the audience. Usually the audience is comprised of the speaker's peers, and the cumulative knowledge of the audi-ence surely will surpass that of the speaker.

In taking an examination, the student will often try to outthink the instructor. As well as the student may think, he can-not know more about the coming examina-tion than the person who has compiled it. The power of positive thinking coupled with the knowledge of understanding the material will allay the buildup of fear and apprehension before the examination. Persons may say that this is simply a state of mind and we are only kidding ourselves. But if it will work, why not use it?

There are other students who believe that their best efforts will not be recog-nized when evaluated against those of others taking the examination. In taking the National Registry Examination the stu-dent is not in competition with anyone except himself. He is not graded against the exceptionally bright. The student is graded on the knowledge that is displayed by his correct answers to the questions.

If this recognition of worth is based upon the evaluation of others who may be cheating during the examination, then worry becomes a fierce reality. The stu-dent must remember that some students will cheat occasionally and others will do it habitually. No examination room can be monitored so completely that cheating is impossible. Cheating has not occurred to a great degree during the writing of the National Registry Examination. If cheating were found, the examination would be taken away and the student re-ported. A student who cheats has little or no respect for either himself or others in his chosen profession. Most times it can be traced to the student who has been doing poorly in the day-to-day class-work. Usually a student who cheats on an examination eventually gets caught in one way or another. In the poor perfor-mance of his daily work, there may arise the question of how he managed to pass the examination. Lack of knowledge is surely the trait of an inadequately trained and questionable student. If a student is truly motivated to become a highly re-spected member of his profession, he has no need or desire to cheat. Perhaps the last sentence is too idealistic, since a book could be written about the devices used by students to take material into an exami-nation with them. If all the time and effort in planning these methods and contrivances were put together in useful study and preparations, what a difference it would make. However, these are the immature students who perhaps fail to be motivated by life or even the courage of their con-victions concerning wrong dealing.

If we could say to the student that this method or that method was the best ap-proach to an examination, it would be so simple. This we cannot do because all of us are individuals. We approach nothing in exactly the same manner. One must search and find his own way, although it be with help.

The student must study and analyze his own personal problem in regard to mental attitudes for examination periods. When it is analyzed, he must proceed with determi-nation to master the art of taking exam-inations. It is too bad that these attributes needed to take examinations are not recog-nized in the early years of high school study and that efforts are not made to cultivate them. It is difficult to accept the fact that courses in "how to study," "note taking," and "speed reading" are all becoming a too familiar part of collegiate life. Yet, how often does one take advantage of them? It is amazing how much the student can learn on his own.

While we have lingered on the element of ridding oneself of fear and substitut-ing a feeling of ease, the element of ade-quate preparation must not be ignored. The knowledge that you have properly and efficiently reviewed the material will bring self-assurance. The inadequate review breeds panic. Self-confidence is always buoyed by knowing you have done your best in providing adequate time and understanding during the review.

Most students have attended high school but upon completion have not learned how to study properly. The study habits of students are to some extent sloppy and distracted. Review sessions consist of constant reading. The solution is to take a course in study habits, but time is valuable.

There are many basic rules on study habits and review. Perhaps now is a good time to enumerate a few and allow you to evaluate your own in the light of them.

PHYSICAL CONDITIONS FOR STUDY

The first condition to consider is environmental. You should have a time and place for study. There should be proper light, heat, ventilation, and furniture. You should seek a quiet place with freedom from distraction. Radios should not be played. Finally, all the materials needed should be close at hand so that you do not have to look for something.

Your physiologic condition as a student plays an important part in the study habits. You need to be obedient to the laws of hygiene. You should seek bodily change and relaxation during long periods of study. Overexertion is as bad as understudy. Stop short of physical fatigue since you remember less and concentrate less as fatigue sets in.

PHYSIOLOGIC CONDITIONS FOR STUDY

The habit of attention to study should be formed, even though it be forced attention. Do not let distractions take your mind from the work. You should concentrate on the task to be performed, having confidence in yourself that it can be done. Remember to avoid the impossible tasks.

Motivation is a must. You should have favorable attitudes, interests, and incentives, as well as definite aims and definite goals in view. The tasks should be related to larger goals. Above all, avoid monotony in study activities.

You need to develop habits. Practiced accurate repetition is always advisable. You should practice reactions that will be useful later. Avoid negative practices; be positive.

You should plan. Everything done at once becomes a jumble of facts, with few related to each other. Distribute periods for study and analyze the tasks. Keep a record of how you spend your time.

The psychologic aspect would not be complete without self-evaluation. Test yourself for the personal characteristics desired. Are you honest in your attempt and aggressive in your approach to study? Do you try to solve problems? You need to note the methods and standards of your work. Does the end result show the result of study?

STUDY HABITS AND PREPARATION

To be prepared one must read. In your reading do you have a purpose, or is your reading just letters on the printed page? Slow readers need to improve their speed and accuracy and at the same time enlarge their vocabularies. While reading you should make mental summaries and formulate questions. Underline the important points. Adapt types of reading—rapid or intensive—to your purpose. Assignments should be first read as a whole and then reread more carefully. Attention should be paid to paragraph headings.

Outlining and note taking are as important as reading. You need to organize the material you read or hear with brief outlines. When possible, construct detailed outlines in light of important points. Take concise notes, utilizing short phrases and abbreviations, when reading and listening to lectures.

Memorization takes its place with the

previous methods. Memorization for memory's sake is useless. It must have a purpose in its relation to what is known and needs to be known. You need to comprehend the material before committing it to memory. Memory work should be distributed in time. Do not do it all at once. Be accurate in the first reading and concentrate during repetitions. Use any device that will help you. Adapt the method, whole or part, to the type of material you are memorizing. To be sure of memory work practice frequent recall and keep a record of your progress.

In problem solving get the problem clearly in mind, collect all the necessary data, and test the hypotheses. When this is complete, evaluate the conclusions.

Reviewing can be time-consuming or concise. It is entirely up to you. The review period will depend upon the attention paid to previously mentioned points. However, review time should be spaced properly, using the notes taken and books to be read. If possible, during review class sessions make outlines and ask questions.

STUDY HABITS AND CLASSROOM PARTICIPATION

The classroom portion of study can be more interesting when you take part in the recitation. Join in the class discussion, but be a good listener also. When in doubt, ask questions. Take adequate yet concise notes.

Pay attention to the lecture and the lecturer's point of view. You should comprehend the important points, evaluating and relating them to your experience.

With the foregoing conditions of study in mind, you may have categorized and examined your study habits in relation to them. Many are easy to understand whereas others need additional explanation. Let us examine three closely interwoven conditions—reading, note taking, and reviewing. Students may believe that every word must be read and in the end may fail to understand the important points. Some students are "underliners"; that is, they try to underline the important passages or key words while they read. This is a good method provided one does not underline everything on the page. Some students tend to commit everything to the pencil and fail to understand the purpose of the method. This method, properly done, allows the student to review the material by scanning the important words or key phrases that have been underlined. An understanding of the subject matter would allow him to write more on the subject during an examination question. A person with a heavily underlined book will have far more reading to do when reviewing for the examination and shows a lack of understanding of the subject matter. The validity lies in whatever method is used to draw attention to those important points on the page or gained from the lecture notes made while in class. Notes copied from another student are of questionable value. Those notes are taken in the light of the other student's understanding.

It is rather remote that any student can copy, word for word, the lecture of any instructor. Even if one could take it down in shorthand, the effort is of little value. Have you ever tried to take notes and draw a diagram at the same time? Admittedly it is difficult. In the stress of continuous shorthand and the blunting of the pencil point, the characters tend to blur together. Thus, one word written may appear as another when reviewed. The allocation of time during review is not compensatory with what is learned. If you must hear the lecture more than once, it would be far better to bring a tape recorder to class and record the lecture in its entirety. The review for such a method is, again, time-consuming. Its good comes from listening and writing down the important points of the lecture for future study.

Another avenue for preparation is to

study the instructor himself. Some teachers use the textbook method of lecture almost exclusively. They follow the material in the book closely, and the student will find outside reading closely allied with their lectures. Some teachers assist the student even more by handing out printed prepared notes. Also there are the teachers who assign reading from one textbook but lecture from additional personal notes. Whatever the method, the student will have to analyze the instructor in the light of it. There are few teachers who enjoy failing a student, but there are some. You will find that most instructors will be honest and explain to you the mechanics of their examination and what to study. They will rely a great deal upon the textbook material since they are sure that the material is covered. Much dissatisfaction exists among students if a question appears on the examination but not in their notes. The cry that the instructor did not cover the subject or point may be used as a whipping point.

What kind of examinations does your instructor give? Are they the same type of examination and questions each time? For example, we had a professor who habitually gave a weekly quiz on the required reading via the true and false methods. His midterm and final examinations were heavily weighed with true-false and multiple-choice questions along with two essay-type questions. The textbook had a required workbook consisting of case histories, problems, and quizzes. It did not take long to note that the weekly quizzes had a familiar ring. Upon investigation it was found that 80% of the weekly quiz questions were verbatim from the workbook examinations. To go further, the bulk of the questions for the midterm and final examinations were derived from this source. Future examinations proved this point. There are many instructors who use the essay-type questions. In constructing an examination these questions are easy to compile. The problem with the essay question is to decide just what the instructor means and what information he wants. The verbose student has nothing to gain by writing page after page of nothing of importance. It does not take an experienced teacher long to notice this practice. The grade is directly proportional to the important material written in the answer.

In the national examination given by the American Registry of Radiologic Technologists, you will find the questions constructed of the multiple-choice method. The questions have beeen submitted over the years by educators, radiologists, and technologists dedicated to the advancement of the profession through education. You may have met many of them. You may only know of them through reputation. You cannot know of their interests and ideas with any degree of accuracy. However, if you have become familiar with other methods of testing, you will find no difficulty with this one.

In our many years as instructors we have often been asked, "Do spelling and neatness count?" We would have to answer that to some extent the grade may be influenced by the spelling. The student would need to know the difference in the meaning of the words "abduct" and "adduct." To incorrectly spell the word in a positioning examination negates the position. Sodium sulfate and sodium sulfite are different chemicals and their properties react to film development in a different manner. Is it important that the spelling be correct? Legible handwriting is a must if one is to express himself correctly. Poor handwriting leads to misinterpretation of words. Most instructors will not take the time to decipher sloppily written answers but will assume that the student is attempting to cover up ignorance. The student's marks will reflect the instructor's attitude.

Many types of questions are used in examinations. Some consist of only one type, whereas others are a composite of many. The examination will be constructed in such a manner as to provide the maximum knowledge of the student and ease in correction. Questions may be posed in the negative as well as the affirmative sense. One of the favorite type questions utilized by instructors is the fill-in, simple completion, or short answer. This type of question consists of short sentences, in each of which one key word is deleted. The "key" word is the one that the student is expected to remember, understand, spell correctly, or interpret. Examples of these follow:

1. The chief danger to the technologist in a radiographic department is exposure to _____.
2. A teleoroentgenogram is taken to decrease _____.
3. The saclike receptacle for the bill is the _____.

These questions are easy to construct and can be taken from any textbook sentence. They will test your recall and knowledge of the subject, and at the same time test your spelling. These questions cannot be corrected by machine.

The objective test scoring, as in true-false questions, is not influenced by outside factors. Except for carelessness, there is no variation in the scores obtained. The danger to the student in taking a test of this nature is to read into the question situations that do not exist. The question must be read at face value and understood only as it is written. If this is remembered, the question becomes reasonable. Some examples of the true-false questions are as follows:

(T) F 1. A film can be tested for radiation fog by processing it without first exposing it.
(T) F 2. Chemical fog is produced by prolonged development.
T (F) 3. The emulsion of an x-ray film contains silver nitrate.

Of all the objective-type questions, the true-false are usually considered the easiest

to make. A good true-false question, which is neither obvious nor ambiguous, is not too easy to make. Since the guessing factor of a true-false test is 50 percent, the scoring formula is often designed to correct for the possibility of guesswork by deducting extra points for all wrong answers, with a lesser deduction for all unanswered ones.

To a student used to taking true-false examinations, questions requiring an obvious reply are quickly answered. For example, questions that use the words *always* and *never* are usually answered as false. Those that contain the expressions *maybe* or *sometimes* may be answered true. By immediately going through a test and eliminating these questions, examination time is cut down. Examples of this are as follows:

1. The only factor affecting contrast is kilovoltage.
2. All x-ray film develops at 68° F.
3. In making a radiograph of the occiput of the skull, a caudad angle of 20 degrees may be used.

In the first question, although we know that kilovoltage is the primary factor affecting contrast, there are many others that also affect to a lesser degree. Therefore, the question could only be false. Processing of films has a varied temperature of development, even in automatic processors, so that the question relating to development must be false. A Towne's view of the occiput calls for an angle of 35 degrees caudad, but it is known from positioning technique that this is not always possible. Sometimes we combine the angle of the tube and the angle of the film to get the desired results. Therefore, the answer to question 3 must be true.

If the answer to a true-false question is not known, should the student guess? As previously stated, it would depend upon the method of correcting. Testing experts advocate the deduction of points for those answered incorrectly and unanswered. In the Registry examination the student is urged to guess at all questions to which he is not sure of the answer. No punishment points are taken from the total score for incorrectly answered questions. It is in one's favor to attempt the answer.

The multiple-choice question is, again, a recognition type of question. The question is constructed with a main question (stem) and a choice of answers (distractors). The question is best constructed by having either a four- or five-part answer. All the choices should be plausible, but only one possible. The four-part answer gives the students only a 25-percent chance of guesswork and the five-part a 20-percent chance. This type of question allows the prepared student to advance more rapidly through the examination. The statement that introduces each question may be in the form of a direct question or a sentence requiring completion.

It is important that in the incomplete sentence the stem makes a complete sentence when combined with the correct answer in the distractors. Most testers agree that the four-part question is as valid as the five-part. Some examples of the multiple choice are as follows:

1. The amount of electrical current flowing in a conductor is measured in:
   (a) watts
   (b) ohms
   (c) amperes
   (d) volts
2. In making a PA radiograph of the abdomen the patient is placed in:
   (a) supine position
   (b) prone position
   (c) decubitus position
   (d) lateral position

Another questioning method used in the National Registry Examination is the matching question. This question contains two lists, one of which is longer than the other. The idea is to match the word in one column with that word most closely related in the other column. Examples of this are as follows:

(a)	anterior	6	1. outside
(b)	superior	3	2. away from
(c)	internal	7	3. upper
(d)	external	1	4. close to
(e)	posterior	8	5. lower
(f)	proximal	4	6. front
			7. inside
			8. back

Examinations properly fashioned will serve a genuine purpose for evaluating the student, the teacher, the teaching effectiveness, and the worth of the system. Modern, functional examinations, which utilize problem solving, critical analysis, and interpretation, are highly desirable both as examination and as teaching procedures. The uses of, reasons for, and real values in examinations are apparent to competent analysts of learning situations. Testing is as necessary in education as accounting is in business. The person who wishes to succeed will use all practice examinations to the fullest. In examinations the easiest questions should be answered first. Do not linger over those of which you are not sure. Leave them until last.

Let us remind you that this book is intended to be nothing more than a review book. It is hoped that it will more carefully prepare you for the writing of your Registry examination. The questions are not formulated to correspond to those of the Registry, but the subject matter is material that should be beneficial to persons taking the National Registry Examination.

3 ETHICS

Ethics refers to the science of human behavior or to systematized principles of morally correct conduct. The science of human behavior can assume many shapes, and each segment of our society dictates its own behavior. In the medical profession there has evolved through the years a system of ethics that is observed and practiced by all those in the medical family. Being in the medical profession we have undertaken the responsibility and duties necessary to assure the health and well-being of those we serve.

Invariably the people with whom we deal are in different stages of ill health, which creates in each of them a different outlook. They become anxious, nervous, and quite often impatient. The afflicted require our immediate and wholehearted services to assist in their quick relief and recovery. We should always be courteous, efficient, fast, and accurate.

Patients quite often will, after seeing you for a while and gaining confidence in you, confide their innermost thoughts. Never should a confidence, disease, diagnosis, or prognosis of a patient be discussed with outsiders or even with persons in related medical areas unless it has some worthwhile bearing on the treatment and eventual cure of the patient. As technologists, it is our responsibility to radiograph the anatomic parts desired, but a technologist never should attempt to interpret the radiographs or discuss the findings with the patient or within the hearing of the patient. Even discussing an unrelated case within the hearing of the patients often will be mistaken and misinterpreted as being about them.

When dealing with patients always speak in a clear, concise manner and explain in detail what you are about to do and the assistance you expect from them. This will not only aid in relaxing the patient, but also cause him to place trust in you. This combination will be valuable in completing the examination. To have to repeat an examination because of an uncooperative patient is inexcusable. Unless the patient is unable to cooperate because of physical or mental conditions, a few minutes spent explaining the procedure is time well used. Repeats not only consume time and talent and increase radiation to the patient, but also reflect poorly on the technologist.

These ethical practices have been tried over the years and, as systematized principles of morally correct conduct, have been found beneficial and correct. Observe them, practice them, and the ethics will have been followed. These are not written laws but have evolved through the years and are accepted.

ETHICS AND HISTORY
Who is a recognized radiologist?

A recognized radiologist is a medical doctor who has specialized in radiology and has passed his board examinations or who by experience has accomplished the equivalent to having passed the board.

Who passes on the qualifications of the radiologist?

The American Board of Radiology is one of the national qualifying specialty boards. It is composed of outstanding practicing radiologists and teachers. Its purpose is to judge the satisfactory completion of training of the candidates.

In what fields may a radiologist entering practice specialize?

The qualified radiologist may become one of the following:

radiologist one who is qualified in the use of x-rays, radium, and radioactive material for diagnosis and treatment of disease

roentgenologist one who is qualified in the use of x-rays only for the treatment and diagnosis of diseases

diagnostic roentgenologist one who is qualified in the use of x-rays only for diagnosis

radiation therapist one who is qualified in the use of x-rays, radium, and radioactive material for treatment only

To whom do radiographs belong?

The radiograph is considered to be part of the patient's hospital record and therefore belongs to the hospital or private office.

May radiographs be loaned?

Yes. Radiographs may be loaned upon a legitimate request, provided the request is in accordance with the hospital and departmental policy. A record should be kept of where films were taken, to whom they were loaned, and the number of films taken.

Under what circumstances would the technologist discuss the diagnostic results of a patient's examination with other hospital personnel?

Under ordinary circumstances results are not discussed with other hospital personnel. The information disclosed by the examination is confidential and should be discussed only with the doctors involved.

What would be the technologist's procedure if a person strange to him and the department requests the loan of a patient's films?

The person should be politely refused, at the same time explaining the regulations of the department. He should be referred to the head of the department for permission to have the films.

Under what circumstances should a technologist diagnose a film?

The right to diagnose films is restricted to those persons who by virtue of experience, knowledge, qualification, and recognition are allowed to practice medicine. There are in existence programs for the preparation of persons with education and experience less than that possessed by the physician but that will qualify them to function as assistants to the physician. This new position will allow others (qualified to a higher degree than technologists) to perform fluoroscopic examinations, interpret films, and administer injections. They will assume duties and responsibilities that the radiologist will delegate, dependent upon the competency of the individual.

What should be done if a patient's relative is anxious to discuss the patient's condition?

It would depend upon what was to be discussed. If the relative is seeking information as to the physical condition of the patient and treatment of this condition, the relative should be referred to the attending physician or the radiologist.

A patient arrives upon the floor with a verbal request for an x-ray examination of a visibly injured part. However, the written request calls for an uninjured part to be x-rayed. What should be done?

Whereas it is not the prerogative of the technologist to determine what part is to x-rayed, this contraindication request should be shown to the radiologist. If possible, the physician requesting the examination should be contacted and the situation discussed. In the absence of all superior personnel the technologist may expose both extremities on a single film without adding radiation exposure to the examination.

A patient is referred to a technologist for a roentgenogram of a particular part. He states that something else is hurting and requests that an x-ray film be taken of the additional part. What should be done?

The technologist should explain to the patient that he is unable to film the part requested since he is bound by the doctor's request. However, he will contact the doctor and ask if the additional examination should be done. If the attending physician is not there, the radiologist should be asked to speak to the patient.

An examination, as a result of technical difficulties, has to be repeated. The technologist does not wish to admit his mistake. What should he do?

If a circumstance like this happens, technologists often place the blame for the repeat upon the patient by telling him that he moved. The psychologic impact of such a statement upon the patient is grave, for it leaves a feeling of insecurity with the patient as to whether he was doing his best to cooperate for the examination. It is no disgrace to the technologist in admitting the fault of the technique.

If a patient is not properly prepared for an x-ray examination, would the technologist criticize the patients' ward personnel for this?

No. Criticism of the patient's ward personnel is certainly not in the realm of good technology. The technologist is not aware of the problems on the ward or of problems, if any, with the patient. Criticism of personnel leads to feelings of insecurity on the part of the patient and to poor public relations.

If a patient asks the technologist for a diagnosis of the films that he has just taken, what should he do?

The technologist should explain to the patient that the training and experience necessary to diagnose films does not belong to him and suggest that the patient discuss it with his attending physician.

What should the technologist's reply be to a patient who criticizes another x-ray department?

The technologist should not criticize another department. He should explain to the patient that he is not informed as to the procedures in the other department.

When may a radiologic technologist own x-ray equipment?

The radiologic technologist should never own x-ray equipment. The conditions for registration by the American Registry of Radiologic Technologists state this.

If a patient asks the purpose of an examination that is being performed, should the technologist give him the clinical information on the requisition?

No. The clinical information on the requisition is for the radiologist to assist him in diagnosing the film. The patient should be instructed to ask his attending physician.

What are some characteristics that a qualified technologist should have or acquire?

Compassion for the other person, whether he be mentally or physically ill

Patience with which to cope with problems that arise, especially those concerning ill patients

Understanding to see the other person's side

Ability to change with the progress of the profession; *to make decisions* that affect the examination and operation of the examination

Neatness in dress and manner

Cheerfulness to the point of contagiousness; to instill this in others even when procedures seem to go wrong

Pleasing personality to enable himself to get along with others

Ability to communicate with others' ideas for work betterment; to be receptive to ideas of others

Thirst for knowledge, which will lead him to the fields of research and technologic writing for the advancement of his profession

While visiting another hospital, unethical conduct is noticed in the x-ray department; to whom should this be reported?

No one. The operation of another x-ray department is not a technologist's affair. He should just make sure that none of this is happening in his own department.

Under what circumstances would the technologist prescribe x-ray treatment?

The technologist should never prescribe x-ray treatment for any disease. This decision is left entirely to the medical staff.

Who discovered x-rays and when?

Wilhelm Conrad Roentgen discovered x-rays on November 8, 1895.

Under what circumstances did Roentgen discover x-rays?

The discovery of x-rays was accidental. Roentgen was experimenting with a glass tube with wiring in it. An induction coil was connected to the tube and current passed into the tube. In this darkened room

a faint greenish light was seen to appear on a nearby bench. Since this was not part of the experiment, another current was passed into the tube. Again the luminescence appeared. Roentgen's search for the material found a cardboard coated with a chemical that would phosphoresce when struck by some form of energy. Repeated exposures with this cardboard about the room showed again and again the faint glow of light.

When did Roentgen report this new discovery?

On December 28, 1895, Professor Roentgen sent his paper, "On a New Kind of Ray," to the Wurzburg Physical Medical Society for publication in its journal.

When was the first public demonstration of x-rays given?

On January 23, 1896, Roentgen gave his first public lecture about this new discovery. At the conclusion of this lecture he asked the anatomist of the university, Albert von Kolliker, if he might x-ray his hand. With permission given by Kolliker the tube was energized while the anatomist's hand was placed upon a photographic film. The processed film showed the bones and soft tissues of the hand.

What reward did Roentgen receive for his discovery of x-rays?

Roentgen realized very little financial reward from his discovery. He belonged to that group of scientists who study for pleasure and whose research delves into the mysteries of nature. However, in 1901 Wilhelm Conrad Roentgen was awarded the Nobel Prize in physics for his discovery of the x-ray.

Was Roentgen the first to discover x-rays?

Roentgen is credited with the actual discovery of x-rays, but much work had actually been performed by others prior to Roentgen's era that prepared the way by providing the equipment used by Roentgen to produce and observe radiation effects. Some individuals and their works that contributed to the discovery of x-rays are as follows (for the sake of brevity confined to the eighteenth century): Michael Faraday in 1838 produced an electrical discharge through space. William Hittorf in 1869 described cathode rays and referred to the passage of electric currents in a vacuum. William Crooks produced vacuum tubes in 1877 and concluded from his observations that cathode rays were in actuality particles carrying negative charges because they were deflected by an electromagnetic field and possessed the ability to heat bodies with which they collided.

One can only conjecture as to the first discoverer of x-rays. It is probably true that many scientists produced x-rays in their experimental work. It is a fact that A. W. Goodspeed of Philadelphia had actually, although accidentally, made a photograph using x-rays on February 22, 1890. The true significance of this photograph was not noted until Roentgen made his announcement to the world. It remained for Roentgen to discover, investigate, and recognize its significance.

Who were the first radiologic technologists (x-ray technicians)?

The first x-ray technicians were medical doctors who had the interest in this new speciality and had the equipment to produce x-rays.

What conditions led to the establishment of the profession of radiologic technologists (x-ray technicians)?

During World War I the use of x-rays focused attention on itself. The use of x-rays for diagnostic studies was increased. Because of all this new application in the use of x-rays and the diagnosis of films, radiologists soon found that they were too busy and were forced to train persons who could produce radiographs.

When did the United States government enter into this new field of x-ray?

Although records and history are a bit hazy, it is known that the use of x-rays by the United States government took place during the Spanish-American War of 1898. It was the first application by any of the military and was used primarily to locate bullets and assist in their removal.

4 MEDICAL TERMINOLOGY

What does medical terminology mean?

Medical terminology is a composite of word roots with prefixes and suffixes that have special meaning for use in a specialized field.

What is a suffix?

A suffix is an abstract element at the end of a word serving derivative, formative, or inflational functions. For example, the word *appendix* refers to the vermiform appendix. If the suffix *itis* were added, the word *appendicitis* would now mean an inflammation of the vermiform appendix.

What is a prefix?

A prefix is one or more letters or syllables combined or united with the beginning of a word to modify its significance. For example, the prefix *hypo-* can mean a deficiency. If we add this prefix to the word *extension*, the new word is *hypoextension* and means a deficiency in the straightening of the part.

Listed below are common prefixes used in medical terminology. Check your understanding of their meaning.

a-, an-	absence of
ab-	off, away from
ad-	to, toward
adeno-	gland
amphi-	upon both sides

angio-	blood vessel
anti-	opposite of
apo-	off, away, implying separation
arterio-	artery
bi-	two, twice
bio-	life
broncho-	bronchus
cardio-	heart
cephalo-	head
cerebro-	brain
chole-	gallbladder
cholang-	biliary ducts
chondro-	cartilage
con-	together, along with
costo-	ribs
cysto-	bladder
derma-	skin
di-	twice, double
dia-	through, apart
dys-	difficult, painful
ec-, ex-, ecto-	out, outside, away from
en-, em-	in, within
endo-	innermost, within
entero-	intestines
epi-	upon, above
gastro-	stomach
hemo-	blood
hetero-	opposite
hydro-	water
hyper-	excessive
hypo-	under, deficient
hystero-	uterus
in-	within, into
infra-	beneath
inter-	between
intra-	inside of
leuko-	white
macro-	abnormally large
mal-	ill, bad

meta-	beyond
micro-	abnormally small
mono-	single
multi-	many
myelo-	brain marrow, spinal cord
myo-	muscle
necro-	dead
neo-	new, recent
nephro-	kidney
neuro-	nerve
ob-, oc-	in front of, against
odonto-	tooth
ortho-	normal
osteo-	bone
pan-	all, universal
para-	beside or apart from
patho-	disease
peri-	about or around
pneumo-	lungs, air
poly-	many
pre-	before
pseudo-	false
pulmo-	lung
pyo-	pus
retro-	in a backward manner, behind
semi-	half
sub-	beneath
super-	excess of, above
supra-	above, upon
trans-	across, through

Listed below are common suffixes. Check your understanding of their meaning.

-agra	seizure of acute pain
-atresia	imperforate
-cele	tumor, swelling
-ectomy	excision
-graph	record
-ism	nature of the word
-itis	inflammation
-lysis	separation
-oma	tumor of
-opia	eye
-osis	disease or process
-otomy	surgical removal of a portion or a part
-scopy	visual examination
-stomy	surgical operation in which a passage is formed
-tomy	incision

The following are general medical and radiologic terms. Knowledge of their meaning and implication makes for a more efficient technologist.

abduct to draw away from midline

abscess a localized collection of pus in a cavity

acetabulum cup-shaped socket in the hip bone receiving the head of the femur

achondroplasia a bone disease in which the cartilage is not properly replaced by bone

acoustic pertaining to the sense of hearing

acrania congenital lack of cranial bones

acromegaly a disease of the pituitary gland producing an overgrowth of bone

acromion outer end of the spine of the scapula

adduct to draw toward the midline

adenoma tumor with glandlike structure

adenopathy disease of the glands

adipose fat stored in the cells of connective tissues

agenesia failure of a body part to develop

alimentary referring to the tubular, food-carrying passage extending from the mouth to the anus

alveolar process bony process supporting the teeth

anastomosis a communication between two vessels

anesthesia suspension of feeling in part of the body

aneurysm abnormal pouching of blood vessel

angioma a tumor composed of blood or lymph vessels

ankylosis abnormal lack of motion and fusion of bone

anomaly marked deviation from standard development

anterior front part of body

anthracosis a disease of the lungs contracted from prolonged inhalation of fine particles of coal dust

antrum a cavity or chamber especially within the bone

apex top

apophysis a process of bone that has

never been entirely separated from the bone of which it forms a part

appendicitis inflammation of the vermiform appendix

appendicular pertaining to the limbs or vermiform appendix

aqueous a watery consistency

arachnoid middle fibrous layer of the meninges covering the brain

arteriography radiographic examination of the arteries

arteriole a minute artery

arteriosclerosis a hardening of the arteries

arthritis inflammation of a joint

articular relation to a joint

articulation place of union of two or more bones

aspirate to remove or draw off by suction

asthma a spasmodic condition of the respiratory tract causing extreme respiratory difficulty

atelectasis collapse of the lung

atresia absence or closure of a body opening

atrium upper chamber of the heart

atrophic wasted

atrophy wasting away of anatomic part caused by lack of nutrition

atypical unusual type

auricular pertaining to the ear or to an auricle

axial along the axis of a part

axilla cavity beneath the junction of the arm and the shoulder; the armpit

benign not malignant, of a mild nature

bicipital groove a furrow located between the two tuberosities of the humerus

bifid cleft or forked

bifurcate divided

bilateral both sides

blastomycosis a fungous infection

bregma point on the surface of the skull at the junction of coronal and sagittal sutures

bronchiectasis saccular dilation of the bronchi

bronchitis inflammation of the bronchi

broncholithiasis calculi in the bronchi

bronchostenosis a narrowing of the bronchus

bursa a calcification situated in the tissues, especially in joint spaces

bursitis inflammation of the bursa

calcicosis pneumonia produced by extended inhalation of calcium dust

calcification deposit of calcium salts in tissue and commonly in bone

callus osseous material exuded around the fragments of a broken bone, ultimately converted into true bone

calvaria cranium

cancellous bone spongy portion of the ends of long bones

cancer malignant new growth of cells

canthus corner on each side of the eye where the upper and lower eyelids meet

capsule enveloping membrane or saclike structure

carcinoma a malignant tumor of epithelial origin

cartilage substance attached to articular bone surfaces

caudad toward the feet or lower end of body

cephalad toward the head or upper part of body

cerebrum the main portion of the brain occupying the upper part of the cranium

cholecystitis inflammation of the gallbladder

cholecystolithiasis the presence of gallstones in the gallbladder

chondritis inflammation of the cartilage

chondroma a benign cartilaginous tumor

chronic slow onset, mild

colostomy an operation that forms an artificial opening in the colon

coma a state of complete loss of consciousness

comminuted splintered, crushed

condyle a round or knucklelike process of a bone, usually for articulation *configuration* general form of a body

congenital present at birth

congestion excessive collection of blood in an organ or tissue

consolidation solidification of a porous structure

constriction narrowing of an opening or tube

contrast media a substance introduced into the body to render radiographic visualization of the part

coracoid process hooklike projection of the scapula

coronal plane frontal plane or plane parallel to the body separating the body into anterior and posterior portions

coronoid fossa depression located on the anterior distal surface of the humerus

coronoid process a bony prominence near the proximal end of the ulna

cortex outer layer of an organ as distinguished from its inner substance

costal relating to the ribs

cranial pertaining to the skull

crest a prominent ridge

cutaneous relating to the skin

cyanosis deficiency of oxygen in the blood resulting in a bluish appearance of the skin

cyst an encapsulated collection of fluid

cystitis inflammation of the urinary bladder

decubitus position in lying down; a bedsore

dermoid resembling the skin

deviate to turn away from

diagnosis art of distinguishing one disease from another

diaphragm musculomembranous partition that separates the abdomen from the thorax

diastole dilation stage of the heart

dilation enlargement of a part or tube

distal distant or remote from the point of origin

distention enlargement of part or condition of body

distortion untrue shape of image

diverticulum a pouch or sac branching off from a cavity or canal

dorsal back surface

dorsum same as posterior, opposed to anterior

ecchymosis escape of blood into surrounding tissue

ectopic abnormal place or position

edema an abnormal presence of fluid in the intercellular tissue spaces

edentulous without teeth

effusion abnormal collection of fluid in body cavity

emphysema distention of the tissues by air in the interstices

empyema pus in the pleural cavity

encroachment invasion of one tissue by another

endocardium lining of the heart cavities

endosteum the layer of vascular connective tissue lining the medullary cavities of bones

erosion destruction along the edge of a structure

etiology cause of a disease

eversion outward rotation of part

evert to turn outward

exostosis an outgrowth of bone

extend to straighten out

extension straightening of the part

external on the outside

extravasation escaping of fluid into the surrounding tissues

fibroma a benign tumor of fibrous tissue

fistula a false tube often leading to a cavity

flaccid flabby

flatus gas in the intestine

flexion act of bending

flexure a turn, bend, or fold

foramen a passageway in the bone

fossa a hollow depression in the bone

fracture a break in the bone

fusion bony union between the epiphysis and diaphysis of the bone

gangrene putrefaction of soft tissue

gastric pertaining to or situated near the stomach

glabella smooth prominence between the eyebrows

glands organs that produce a particular substance to be used in or eliminated from the body

gonads sex glands

hamulus any hook-shaped process

hepatic pertaining to the liver

hiatus a cleft

hilus a depression or pit at that part of an organ where the vessels and nerves enter

idiopathic disease of unknown origin

ileus obstruction of small intestine

inferior below

inguinal pertaining to the groin

intercostal between the ribs

inversion inward rotation

irradiation therapeutic application of ionizing radiation

junction the point of joining or uniting

kyphosis curvature of the spine with convexity backward producing a humpback

lamina flattened part of either side of the arch of the vertebra

lateral away from the midline toward the side

lingual pertaining to the tongue

lobe a part of an organ demarcated by globular shape

lordosis curvature of the spine with convexity forward

lumen a channel of a tubular structure

luxation abnormal slipping of one part on another at a joint space

malignant of severe nature; tending to go from bad to worse

meatus the opening at the end of a canal

medial being situated or occurring in the middle of the body

mediastinum the middle compartment of the chest containing all of the thoracic viscera except the lungs

meninges the lining of the spinal canal and cranial cavity

mental pertaining to the mind, chin, or lower jaw

mesentery the fold by which intestines are attached to the posterior wall of the abdominal cavity

matastasis transfer of a disease from one region to another by lymphatics or bloodstream

mucosa mucous membrane

mucus secretion of the mucous membrane

myeloma a tumor of the bone marrow

myocardium heart muscle

necrosis destruction of a tissue

neoplasm a new growth or tumor

nephritis inflammation of the kidney

nephroptosis dropping of the kidney from normal position

neuritis inflammation of the nerves

oblique a semilateral position

obliterate to remove completely

obturator foramen oval opening in the lower portion of the pelvis near the hip joint

occlusion closing of a part of the body

opacity an object impervious to radiation

opaque impervious to light rays

oral pertaining to the mouth

orifice an opening

osseous system the bony skeleton

ossicle a tiny bone

osteoma a benign bone tumor

ovum the female reproductive cell

palmar referring to palm of hand

paralysis loss of nerve control of muscles

parenchyma functional parts of an organ as opposed to its framework

parietal lateral or outer aspect

pathology science that deals with the nature and cause of disease

perforation breaking through a part, tearing

pericardium membranous sac containing the heart

periosteum fibrous covering of the bone

periphery outer portion of the part

peristalsis contraction movement of the part by which contents are propelled along

peritoneum serous membrane lining the

abdominal wall and investing the viscera

phrenic pertaining to the diaphragm; pertaining to the mind

plantar relating to the sole of the foot

pleurisy inflammation of the pleura

pneumothorax air in the pleural cavity

polyp smooth growth from a mucous surface of the body attached by a stem

posterior situated behind or toward the rear

process any marked prominence or projecting part

pronation ventral side down, face down

protuberance that which bulges behind the surrounding or adjacent surface

proximal near the source of origin

ptosis sagging of an organ from its normal position

pulmonary pertaining to the lungs

radioactive property of spontaneous emission of radiation

radioisotope radioactive forms of chemicals

radiolucent permitting partial penetration by x-ray

radiopaque not permitting penetration by radiation

ramus a branch or primary division

renal pertaining to the kidney

sagittal center of body, straight

sarcoma an abnormal rapid growth of tissues, usually of a malignant nature

scoliosis lateral curvature of the spine

sella turcica a saddlelike bone structure at the base of the skull that shelters the pituitary gland

septum a partition

sinus a tract in soft tissue with external opening; a natural air cavity in a bone

spasm involuntary contraction of muscle

specific gravity ratio of the weight of a given volume of liquid or solid substance to the weight of an equal volume of water

sphincter a muscle structure encircling an orifice

spina bifida a defect of the neural arch

spondylitis inflammation of one or more vertebrae

spondylolisthesis forward luxation of the vertebra on the sacrum

stenosis a constriction of the lumen or opening of a canal

superior above, higher

supination turning upward

supine lying on the back

surface dose dose of radiation given to the surface of the part and measured in roentgens

suture a line of union between bones of the skull

symphysis line of union of two distinct bones

syndrome a complex of symptoms

systole contractive stage of heart

tangential touching at a single point

therapy used in radiology to indicate the treatment of disease with radium and x-rays

thorax pertaining to the chest

thrombus clotting of blood within a vessel

tolerance dose of x-rays a dose of x-rays that will be tolerated by the skin without injury

transverse lying crosswise

trauma an injury or wound

trochanter a very large process below the neck of the femur

tubercle a small rounded projection of a bone

tuberosity a large rounded projection on a bone

tumor a mass of new tissue that grows independently of its surrounding structures and performs no physiologic function

ventral anterior surface

vertex top of the head

vesicle a small sac containing fluid

viscus an internal organ enclosed within a cavity

volar relating to palm or sole

The following are specific terms pertinent to physics and radiologic technique.

acceleration rate of change of motion or action

accessory additional or supplementary

actinic that portion of light that affects a photographic emulsion

adjustable resistance a resistance whose value may be adjusted

air dielectric value of air as a dielectric is taken as 1, and the value of other dielectrics are based on a comparison with the value of air

air dose dose of radiation measured in roentgens in free air

air gap air space between the ends of conductors

air insulation use of air as an insulator, with or without additional insulation of other materials

alloy a metal composed of two or more metals

alpha particle a positively charged particle emitted from the nucleus of certain radioactive elements

alternating current (AC) time-rate of flow of electric charge periodically, first in one direction and then in the opposite direction

alternating current generator a generator producing alternating currents

alternating current instruments instruments that measure or record the various values of alternating currents such as voltage, amperage, phase, and frequency

alternating current rectifier a device for changing alternating current into direct current by electric, mechanical, or chemical action

alternations one-half cycle of an alternating current

alternator a generator that produces an alternating current

ambient temperature the temperature of the air or other medium surrounding the heated parts of an electric device

American wire gauge (AWG) the gauge generally adopted and used for measuring the size of wires in the United States

ammeter an instrument that measures and indicates the number of amperes flowing in an electric circuit

ammeter shunt a low-resistance conductor placed in parallel with an ammeter so that the greater part of the measured current flows through the shunt, only a small part of the total flow going through the ammeter itself

amperage strength of an electric current in amperes

ampere steady current that deposits silver at the rate of 0.001118 gram per second from a solution of nitrate of silver in water—is taken as a unit of current; it has been computed that 1 ampere of current corresponds to a flow of 6.25×10^{18} electrons per second, that is, 6.25 billion billion electrons per second

ampere hour a measure of quantity of electricity; the quantity that flows through a circuit in 1 hour when the flow is 1 ampere

angstrom unit a unit of length usually reserved for expressing wave length; 1 angstrom equals 10^{-8} cm.

anion a negatively charged ion

anneal to soften by heating and allowing to cool slowly

area of conductor size of a section through a conductor, usually measured in circular mils

armored cable conductor cable having a woven or spirally wound metallic covering over its insulation so that it is protected against mechanical injury

artificial magnet a manufactured permanent magnet

atom smallest part of an element; it consists of a nucleus, composed (with the exception of hydrogen) of a number of protons and neutrons and of an extranuclear portion composed of electrons equal in number to the nuclear protons

atomic number integer that expresses the

positive charge of the nucleus in multiples of the electronic charge

atomic structure a theory that matter is composed of a vast number of particles, or atoms, bound together by a force of attraction

atomic weight weight of one atom of an element as compared to the weight of an atom of hydrogen; one atomic weight unit is equal to 1.660×10^{-24} grams

attraction effect between magnetized bodies or between a magnet and iron or steel by which they are drawn together

autotransformer a transformer in which the primary and secondary are combined

ballistic meter an ammeter having a weighted needle used to measure milliampere second—the product of milliamperes and time (in seconds)

battery a group of cells or often a single cell producing an electric current

beta particle a negatively charged particle that is emitted from the nucleus of certain radioactive elements

Bucky diaphragm (Potter-Bucky diaphragm) a device used in radiography consisting of a grid of lead strips so arranged as to reduce the effect of secondary radiation on a radiograph

bus bar a heavy rod or bar of copper carrying one of the main circuits on a switchboard or between distributing points

cable a conductor composed of a number of separate conductors

calibrate to compare the reading of a measuring instrument with some fixed standard or with another instrument

calibration (x-ray) determination of the kvp value of each autotransformer tap at various milliamperages, checking these values by means of sphere-gap or a prereading voltmeter

capacitance inherent property of an electric circuit that opposes any change in voltage in the circuit; also defined as "the property of a circuit whereby energy may be stored"

capacitor a device for holding and storing charges of electricity

capacity used in electricity to indicate the full extent to which a condenser can be charged; often used to indicate an actual charge on any electrode

cardboard holder a light-tight film container made of heavy cardboard and paper used in radiography

cassette a light-tight film holder usually containing a pair of intensifying screens used in radiography

cathode negative terminal of an electrical apparatus

cathode ray a stream of electrons leaving the cathode in a discharge tube

cation positive ion

centigrade a scale for the recording of temperature with freezing at 0° C. and boiling at 100° C. (distilled water at sea level)

central ray the center of the beam of x-rays coming from an x-ray tube

characteristic radiation secondary radiation typical of a given element

choke coil a coil having high inductance but low ohmic resistance used in a circuit to limit the flow of current

cinefluorography the process wherein motion pictures are produced of the images appearing on a fluorescent screen

circuit (electrical) course traversed by an electric current

circuit breaker a form of switch, usually automatic in action, that opens a circuit under abnormal or dangerous conditions

circular mil area of a circle 1/1000 inch (1 mil) in diameter

cohesion force that unites the particles of a body

coil an insulated wire wound in the form of a spiral

collision a close approach of two or more objects (particles, photons, atomic or nuclear systems) during which there occurs an interchange of quantities such as energy, momentum, and charge

compensator a correcting device

compound a substance formed by two or more elements

Compton effect interaction of a photon with matter, wherein a part of the energy of the photon is transferred to an orbital electron of an atom; the photon then proceeds with diminished energy and with altered direction (and hence longer wave length)

condenser see *capacitor*

conductance ease with which a conductor carries an electric current

conductor material in which a current flow is readily established

cone a metallic tubular extension placed between the x-ray tube and the patient to limit the field of examination

constant decay ratio of the radioactivity lost by a material per unit time to the radioactivity of the material

constant dielectric dielectric value of any substance compared with air, which is taken as 1

contrast (radiographic) difference in densities of a radiograph as perceived by the naked eye

convergence coming together of lines or rays

cosmic rays ionizing radiation from outer space with energies as great as 10^{10} to 10^{15} electron volts bombarding the earth and its atmosphere

coulomb practical unit of electric charge; the quantity afforded by an ampere of current in one second flowing against 1 ohm of resistance with a force of 1 volt

counter electromotive force (CMF) a voltage or electromotive force that opposes the normal or impressed voltage in a circuit and sends current in the opposite direction

Crookes' tube a vacuum tube used by Sir William Crookes in early experimental work

curie quantity of radon in equilibrium with 1 gram of radium

current (electric) flow of electrons

cycle one complete wave of an alternating current

d'Arsonval meter a voltmeter or ammeter whose pointer is attached to a wire carried between the poles of a permanent magnet

deenergize to stop current from flowing in an electrical circuit or portion thereof

deflection movement of the indicating pointer of an electric measuring instrument

demagnetization process of magnetism disappearing from a magnet

density (radiographic) relative "blackness" or areas on an x-ray film after exposure to x-ray and processing

depth dose amount of radiation actually being delivered within the tissue being treated

detail clearness in a radiograph of the finer structures

developer (x-ray) solution used for the development of the radiographic image on x-ray film

dielectric strength ability of an insulating material to resist electric potential or voltage

difference of potential difference of voltage or electric pressure between two points

direct current (DC) an electric current flowing always in the same direction

discharge a passage of electricity from a source

dosage rate time rate at which radiation dose is applied

dose amount of radiation delivered at a specific point

double exposure two superimposed exposures on the same film

double focus tube an x-ray tube having two focal spots

double pole (DP) connected to both

sides of a circuit or arranged for connecting into two circuits

double throw switch (DTS) a knife switch whose blades are pivoted at the center of the switch so that a circuit may be completed through either of two paths

dry cell a primary electric cell using carbon and zinc for electrodes

dryer device for drying x-ray film after processing

ductile the property that permits a metal to be drawn into wire

eddy currents currents induced in a mass of conductive material by a varying magnetic field

effective wave length the wave that would produce the same penetration as an average of the various wave lengths in a heterogeneous bundle of rays

efficiency (electric) the ratio of the useful work or output of an electric device to the power supplied to it

electric horsepower the horsepower measured in watts; 746 watts equals 1 electric horsepower

electrode a terminal of a conductor of electricity, usually of metal or carbon

electrolyte any solution that conducts electricity by means of its ions

electromagnet a temporary magnet made by passing an electric current through a coil of wire surrounding a core of soft iron

electromagnetic field the magnetic field produced about an electromagnet

electromagnetic induction (law of) magnetic lines of force, cut at right angles by a conductor or electricity, induce in that conductor an electric current

electromotive force pressure of an electric charge; voltage

electron a small, negatively charged body forming part of the atomic structure

electroscope an instrument for the detection of small charges of electricity

electrostatic static electricity

element substance that cannot be decomposed by the ordinary types of chemical reaction or made by chemical union

emanation (in radiology) a gaseous disintegration product given off from radioactive substance

energize to cause a magnetic material such as a magnet core to become magnetized or magnetic; to send current through a circuit or through a winding or coil

energy capacity for performing work

exit dose an x-ray dose to the skin opposite the irradiated surface

exposure subjection of a photographic film to the effects of light or x-ray

Fahrenheit a scale for the recording of temperature in which the freezing point of water is indicated as 32° and the boiling point as 212°

farad the unit in which electrostatic capacity is measured; the capacity of a condensor that will give a pressure of 1 volt when a current of 1 ampere flows into it for 1 second

field space in which there are magnetic lines of force about a magnet

field coil windings or conductors around the field magnets of generators, motors, and so on

field magnet iron and steel parts through which the field lines of force pass in a generator or motor

field pole one of the ends of the field magnet between which an armature of a generator or motor rotates

filament a fine, threadlike conductor that carries current in an incandescent lamp and that becomes white-hot to give light; also the conductor in a vacuum tube that may be heated to produce a supply of electrons directly or heated to in turn heat a cathode that will produce free electrons

filament control (x-ray unit) a device for regulating the filament temperature of an x-ray tube *filament transformer* a step-down transformer that supplies the current for the x-ray tube filament

film a thin, flexible, transparent sheet of polyester or acetate or similar material coated with a light-sensitive emulsion

filter in x-ray physics a sheet of metal through which the rays pass before striking the object to be examined or treated

filtration (x-ray) the passing of a roentgen ray through certain metals or other materials by which the nonpenetrating or soft rays are removed, only the penetrating or hard rays passing through

fission the dividing of an atom (heavy nucleus) into two approximately equal parts by means of neutron bombardment

fixed resistance a resistance that is not adjustable

fixer solution used in the processing of x-ray film that removes all of the unexposed silver halide crystals and fixes the image onto the film permanently

fluctuating current a current whose voltage and amperage change at irregular intervals while always flowing in the same direction

fluorescence the emission of visible light by a crystal when subjected to an activating source

fluorescent screen a sheet of radiolucent material coated with a crystalline compound that fluoresces when exposed to x-rays

fluoroscope a piece of x-ray apparatus consisting of an x-ray tube properly housed and mounted so that x-rays emanating from the tube strike upon a fluorescent screen

fluoroscopy examination by means of a fluoroscope

flux the magnetism of lines of force flowing through a magnetic circuit (measured in maxwells)

flux density the number of lines of force in a given cross-sectional area

focal-skin distance the distance from the focal spot to the skin of the patient

focal spot the small spot on the target of an x-ray tube from which x-rays are emitted; receives the impact of the electron stream from the cathode

fog a hazy appearance of a radiograph due to exposure to light or x-ray or subjection to unusual chemical action

force that which changes the speed or motion of anything, either to cause motion, to increase or decrease the speed, or to stop motion

frequency (F) the number of cycles per second of an alternating current

fuse a protective device made of wire or strip of fusible metal inserted in a circuit; melts when the current becomes too strong

galvanometer an instrument for measuring small currents or voltage

gamma ray electromagnetic radiation of extremely short wave length emitted by radioactive elements

generator a machine that changes mechanical power into electrical power

grain degree of coarseness of a screen or film emulsion

grid (vacuum tube) a meshwork of wire interposed between the anode and cathode of an electron tube

grid (x-ray device) a device composed of alternate thin strips of lead and a radiolucent material encased in a suitable binder and placed between the patient and the radiographic film to absorb some of the scattered secondary radiation that would otherwise be detrimental if permitted to reach the film

ground (electricity) an electric connection to the earth, either directly or indirectly

grounded circuit a circuit completed through ground, through the earth; because the earth is a good conductor, it prevents the accumulation of electric charges

grounded neutral a grounded, neutral wire in a three-wire circuit

half value layer the thickness of a given material, in addition to the normal working filter, required to reduce x-radiation intensity by 50 percent

heat loss the loss of power due to increased resistance in heated conductors

helix anything having a spiral form (helix of wire)

heterogeneous radiation radiation having several different frequencies or wave lengths

high tension high voltage; voltage of 1,000 or more volts

homogeneous radiation radiation having an extremely narrow band of frequencies or wave lengths

horsepower (HP) the unit in which mechanical or electrical power is measured; 1 horsepower is the power required to raise 33,000 pounds 1 foot in one minute

hot cathode tube (Coolidge tube) any x-ray tube utilizing a heated cathode for its source of electrons

hysteresis the phenomenon in which the magnetism of a sample of iron or steel, produced by a magnetic field, lags behind the field when the field is made to vary through a cycle of values

hysteresis loss the work or power required to reverse the direction of magnetism in iron or steel

image designates in radiography and photography the impression made on an x-ray or photographic film by x-rays or light

impedance (Z) the apparent resistance of an alternating current circuit that is analogous to the actual electrical resistance to a direct current; it is equal to the vector sum of the resistance and the reactance of the circuit

impedance factor the ratio of the alternating current impedance in a circuit to the ohmic resistance in the same circuit

impulse one alternation of an alternating current; one-half cycle

impulse timer an instrument used in radiography for timing fractional second exposures

induced current current caused by mutual or electromagnetic induction

induced electromotive force the electromotive force induced in a conductor by a magnetic field of changing intensity or direction

induced magnetism magnetism produced by the action of electric current or by the action of other magnets

induction appearance of an electric current or of magnetic properties because of the presence of another electric current or magnetic field nearby

induction coil an apparatus for transforming a direct current, such as an ordinary battery current, by induction into an alternating current of high potential

inductor a part of an electric apparatus that acts upon another or is itself acted upon by induction

insulate (electric) to separate from conducting bodies by means of nonconductors or insulators

insulator a dielectric material used to confine or prevent the flow of an electric current

intensifying screen a screen composed of fluorescent material placed in contact with an x-ray film to intensify the action of x-rays in radiography

inverse square law the law that is applied to all point-source radiation; the intensity of illumination is inversely proportional to the square of the distance

ion a charged atom or molecular-bound group of atoms; sometimes also a free electron or other charged subatomic particle *ion pair* positive and negatively charged ions formed by the ionization of a single atom

ionization process wherein ions are produced

ionization chamber an instrument for measuring quantity of radiation as a function of the ionization produced by radiation

iron loss loss of power caused by hysteresis and by eddy currents in the iron cores of electric devices

joule (J) energy expended in one second by an electric current of 1 ampere in a resistance of 1 ohm and is equal to 0.738 foot-pounds

jumper a conductor connected around a part of a circuit, the connection being made for emergency work or test purposes

kenetron a valve tube for rectification of high voltage current

kilovolt unit of electromotive force of potential equal to 1,000 volts

kilovolt-ampere (kva) rating form for alternating current generators (instead of kilowatts); determined by the formula kv × I equals kva

kilovolt-peak (kvp) the crest value in kilovolts of electromotive force or potential of a pulsating source of electric potential

kilowatt a unit equal to 1,000 watts

kilowatt-hour a unit of energy equivalent to the work done by 1 kilowatt in one hour

Kirchoff's law the algebraic sum of the currents that meet at any point of a circuit is zero

lag the period of time elapsing between the application of a stimulus and the resultant reaction

laminated having many thin layers

laminated core a magnetic core made up of thin sheets of iron or special steel bound together into a solid piece, insulated from one another by insulating material

latent image the invisible effect produced on a film by the action of light or x-rays before development

latitude the range of exposure of an x-ray film permissible for a good diagnostic result

leak (electric) a loss of current through a short circuit or an accidental ground

line of force an imaginary line that indicates the direction in which magnetism flows between magnetic poles or around conductors carrying a current or an electric charge

load (electric) the power required to operate current-consuming devices

lodestone a piece of natural magnetic iron ore

Lysholm grid a stationary grid of fine lead strips that is used like a Potter-Bucky diaphragm

magnet a body that will attract magnetic material

magnetic contactor a device operated by an electromagnet to close and open contacts in a circuit

magnetic field the field of magnetic force emanating from a magnet

magnetic induction magnetic flux density in any substance when immersed in a magnetic field

magnetism the ability of an energized coil or a natural magnet to attract particles of magnetizable substances

mass (atomic) measure of the quantity of matter in an element; one atomic mass unit equals 1.657×10^{-24} gm., or 9.31×10^8 electron volts

meter an instrument used for measurement; a measure of length equal to 39.37 inches

mica insulating material

microfarad one millionth of a farad

milliammeter (see *ammeter*)

milliampere one thousandth of an ampere

million electron volt (mev) one million electron volts

millivolt one thousandth of a volt

molecule the smallest quantity of a material that can exist by itself and retain all of the chemical properties of the material

motor (electric) a device for changing electric energy into mechanical energy

motor-generator a transforming device consisting of a motor mechanically connected to a generator

natural radioactivity radioactivity by naturally occurring substances

neutron an electrically neutral or uncharged particle of matter existing along with protons in the atoms of all elements except the hydrogen nucleus

nuclear radiation radiation emitted when changes occur in the nucleus of an atom

nucleus the heavy central part of an atom in which most of the mass and the total positive electric charge is concentrated

ohm a unit of measure of electrical resistance; 1 ohm of resistance will allow 1 ampere of current to flow when 1 volt is applied to the circuit

ohm meter an instrument that measures and directly indicates resistance in ohms

Ohm's law the rule or law stating the relation of the pressure in volts, the current in amperes, and the resistance in ohms in an electric current

oil transformer a transformer that is insulated by a bath of oil; the oil circulates, cooling the heated parts of the transformer while acting as an insulator

opaque impervious to light rays or, by extension, to roentgen rays

open circuit an incomplete circuit; one broken at any point, so that current does not flow through any part of it

overload a load in amperes greater than an electric device or circuit is designed to carry or to operate

paper capacitor a capacitor using paper for its dielectric

parallel circuit several circuits or electric parts so connected that current from a source divides between them

peak voltage the highest voltage attained in a circuit in a given period

penetration the ability of radiation to extend down into and go through substances

permanent magnet a hard alloy that keeps its magnetic strength for long periods of time with little change

permeability the ability of a certain magnetic material to carry magnetic flux of lines of force; a measure of the ease with which the flux is carried; opposed to reluctivity

phase a point or position to which an alternating current wave has increased toward maximum from a position of zero potential; measured in degrees, one complete cycle being divided into 360 degrees

phosphorescence the emission of light by a crystal after the activating source has ceased

photoelectric effect the excitation and ionization of atoms by the interaction of radiant energy

photoelectron an electron emitted in a photoelectric effect

photofluorography the photographic recording of the fluoroscopic images on small films using a fast lens

photographic effect (PE) the effect of light or x-rays on a photographic emulsion

photographic emulsion the emulsion of the halides of silver that form the sensitive coating of a photographic or x-ray film

photon the term applied to a single electron or gamma ray when it is considered as a projectile rather than a wave or ray

phototimer an instrument usually consisting of a photomultiplier tube and associated electronic circuits designed to terminate radiographic exposures automatically

polarity the negative or positive electric charge of a body or terminal

polarization the formation of gases on the plate surfaces in electric batteries; the gases are formed by the electrolyte by electrolytic action and form partial insulators on the plates

pole (electric) the positive or negative terminal of a circuit

pole (magnet) the magnetic pole, designated either north or south

polyphase an alternating current circuit having two or more voltages of the same number of cycles but not in phase with one another

positive charge a charge of electricity wherein a deficiency of electrons exists in a body

potential electromotive force, pressure, or voltage

potential difference the difference in electric pressure or voltages between two points in a circuit

potentiometer an instrument for making accurate comparisons between a known voltage or standard voltage and another voltage

Potter-Bucky diaphragm a piece of radiographic apparatus consisting of a grid of parallel strips of lead arranged on the radius of curvature of a cylinder, the center of which is at the focal spot of the x-ray tube; used to reduce the effects of scattered radiation

power (P) the rate at which work is done, measured in such units as horsepower, foot-pound-seconds, watts, and so on

power loss the power, measured in watts, that disappears in transmitting current through a circuit

primary circuit a circuit connected directly to a source

primary radiation radiation arising directly from the target of an x-ray tube or radioactive source

proton a positively charged particle found in the nucleus of an atom

puncture (electric) a break through an insulator caused by high voltage

rad unit of absorbed dose equal to 100 ergs/gm.

radiant energy that form of energy that is transmitted through space without the support of an apparent media

radiation the projection through space of any form of electromagnetic waves

radiation therapy the use of radiation of any type in the treatment of disease

radiograph a photographic film that has been exposed to x-rays after they have passed through the part to be examined

radiography the science that deals with the taking and interpreting of x-ray films

radiologist a physician who uses all forms of radiation in the diagnosis and treatment of disease

radiology the science that deals with the use of all forms of radiant energy in the diagnosis and treatment of disease

radium a radioactive element used in the treatment of disease

ratio of transformer the ratio of the number of turns in the primary to the number of turns in the secondary of a transformer

reactance the weakening of an alternating current caused by passage through a coil or wire

reciprocal the quotient of unity divided by any quantity

recoil electron an electron ejected from the extranuclear portion of an atom in the process of the Compton effect

rectification (electric) the process of changing alternating current into pulsating direct current

rectifier a device that changes alternating current into unidirectional current by electronic, mechanical, or chemical action

relay (electric) a device for controlling

an electric circuit by opening and/ or closing contacts; the action of the contacts may be activated by a circuit separate from that being controlled

reluctance resistance to the flow of magnetism (measured in oersteds)

repulsion the act of repelling; the force with which bodies, particles, or like forces repel one another

residual magnetism the magnetism that remains in a piece of soft iron when a magnetizing force is removed

resistance (electric) the opposition offered by a substance or body to the passage through it of an electric current (measured in ohms)

resistor (electric) a device having resistance

rheostat a device for regulating a current by means of variable resistance

roentgen (r) a unit of radiologic dose; the quantity of x- or gamma radiation that the associated corpuscular emission per 0.001293 gm. of air produces in air ions carrying one electrostatic unit of electric charge of either sign

roentgen-equivalent-man a unit of dose useful in protection equal to relative biologic effectiveness times absorbed dose in rads (symbol rem)

roentgen-equivalent-physical a unit of absorbed dose equal to 93 ergs/gm.; this unit is now superceded by rad (symbol rep)

roentgen rays x-rays

roentgen therapy x-ray therapy

rotary convertor a motor-generator set that, when operated by one type of current, produces another

rotating anode tube an x-ray tube so constructed that the target rotates or revolves about an axis; the rotating portion of the tube is the rotor of a repulsion-induction motor

safelight a light used in a darkroom to which films may be exposed without fog

saturation (magnetic) the greatest num-

ber of lines of force or flux that a certain magnet or magnetic material will carry

scattered radiation radiation whose direction has been altered by an interaction with an atom

screen lag residual illumination remaining on the screen after the exposure has terminated

secondary electron an electron ejected from an atom as a result of a collision with a charged particle or photon

secondary radiation particles or photons produced in matter by the interaction of a radiation regarded as primary

secondary winding that portion of a transformer in which current is induced

separator a sheet of wood, rubber, or other insulating material placed between the plates of storage battery cells to prevent electric contact between the plates

series circuit a circuit in which all the parts are connected end-to-end so all the current passing through any one part must pass through every other part in the circuit

service wires wires connecting interior circuits of a house or building with the outside supply circuit

sheathing of a cable the outside covering that protects a cable from mechanical injury or from the effects of water, oils, acids, and so on

shell transformer a transformer in which the iron core is built around the outside of the windings

short-stop an acid solution into which the films may be immersed before fixing in order to terminate development

short circuit an accidental connection of low resistance between the two sides of a circuit so that little or no current flows through the current-consuming device in the circuit

shunt one of the current paths in a parallel circuit

skin-dose (therapy) that amount of radiation delivered at the level of the skin

silicon steel steel alloys with silicon; has a low hysteresis and eddy current loss

silver a metal having a lower electric resistance than copper

simple circuit a circuit connecting one source with a current-consuming device

sine wave an alternating current wave formed following the curve of sines; the ideal form of an alternating wave

single phase an alternating current having but one phase; but one wave

single pole switch a switching device having but one contact

solenoid a coil or winding of several layers of conductors that are insulated from each other

space charge the current in a hot cathode tube limiting effect of the electron cloud in the region of the cathode

spectrum result of dispersion of waves of radiation of different wavelengths; for both light and x-ray

speed (x-ray film) the degree of sensitiveness to x-rays of x-ray film

sphere gap a variable gap between the spheres connected across a high tension circuit, the purpose of which is to measure the voltage

split phase currents of different phases obtained from a phase circuit by the use of reactances

stabilizer an instrument used in an x-ray unit to render the milliamperage output of the x-ray tube constant

standard ohm a wire having the resistance of exactly 1 ohm and used for comparison and calibration

static charge a quantity of electricity existing as a charge on conductors or on the plates of a condenser

static electricity electricity at rest, such as in the charge of a condenser, as distinguished from the electric current that is electricity in motion

step-down (transformer) a transformer for reducing voltage

step-up (transformer) a transformer for increasing voltage

storage battery a number of storage cells in a single case and connected with each other to give a desired voltage and current capacity

sulfuric (sulfuric acid) the acid used, when diluted with water, as the electrolyte in the lead-acid storage battery and in other types of electric cells (H_2SO_4)

suppression elimination, as, for example, the suppression of a phase of current by a rectifier

surface leakage leakage of current across the surface of an insulator

surge a rapid increase in voltage

surge impedance the impedance resulting from inductance and capacitance in an alternating current circuit

switch a device for opening, closing, or changing the connection in an electric circuit

symbol a letter or other sign that has been adopted and is understood to stand for some certain value of measure

synchronizer a device for indicating when alternating currents are in phase or synchronous

synchronous motor an alternating current motor whose speed is in proportion to the frequency of the current supply

tachometer an instrument that indicates the speed of rotating parts

target the positive terminal of an x-ray tube, which receives the electrons and emits x-rays

thermoelectron an electron emitted by a heated body, as the filament of an x-ray tube

three-wire circuit an electric circuit in which a neutral conductor is used

time-constant the length of time it takes the current in a circuit to reach a certain value with a given voltage applied to the circuit

timer an instrument used on an x-ray unit to complete the electric circuit so that x-rays will be produced for a limited period of time

transformer a device used to change alternating current from one voltage value to another

transformer efficiency the ratio of the electric power going into a transformer to the power output of the secondary circuit from the transformer

transformer oil the insulating oil used to fill the space around the transformer windings and core

transformer loss the difference between the power input to a transformer and the power output of a transformer

transmission line the conductors through which high voltage is carried for long distances between the power station and the substation

tungsten a very hard metal that resists the effects of arcing and that has a very high melting point

vacuum area devoid of gas

vacuum tube a sealed tube with the contained gas exhausted to a pressure low enough to permit the passage of an electric discharge between metallic electrodes projecting into the tube from the outside; sometimes called a valve or electron tube

variable capacitor a capacitor whose capacitance may be varied

variable inductor the inductance in circuits or coils having an iron core whose permeability changes with the change in magnetomotive force.

variable resistor a resistor whose resistance may be varied

volt (E) the fundamental unit of measure of electrical pressure or electromotive force; defined as the electrical pressure necessary to force 1 ampere of current through 1 ohm of resistance

voltmeter an instrument for measuring electric pressure

watt the practical unit of electric power; 1 watt is the power produced by current or 1 ampere at a pressure of 1 volt

watt-hour a measure of electrical power; 1 watt for one hour

watt-hour meter an instrument for measuring power consumed in watt-hours

Wheatstone bridge a device for measuring a resistance by comparing it with known resistance in the bridge

wire a piece of drawn metal usually used as a conductor

x-ray electromagnetic radiations or vibrations (photons) emitted when high-speed electrons strike orbital electrons

x-ray tube a vacuum tube used for the production of x-rays

zero potential having neither positive nor negative electric potential

5 MEDICAL AND SURGICAL DISEASES

Since the discovery of x-rays, the possibilities to be derived from them in diagnosing and treating diseases were recognized. The possibilities have proved to go beyond the expectations of the early pioneers. We have, of course, learned more about the properties and nature of these invisible rays than was possible for the early scientist to learn. Although tremendous progress has been made in the use of x-rays, there is still much to be learned. The diseases that have been conquered have not reduced the total number of diseases since new ones are being discovered or recognized. X-rays have proved to be of immeasurable assistance in the diagnosis and treatment of diseases and in the future will add to the store of knowledge already gained.

Diseases of one type or another have been present since the origin of man and have presented challenges that man has been trying to overcome in the never-ending search for better health and longer life expectancy. The term "disease" is defined as "the impairment of the normal state of the living animal or plant body" that affects the performance of the vital functions. The term normal state is itself confusing since no single definition can adequately cover the many variations. It is possible to observe the effective function of two or more organs that in appearance might be different although each can per-

form the assigned task. Disease might further be defined as the impairment of expected functions and responses to certain given stimuli and situations; diseases of this type may assume a variety of pathologic forms. It will be noted that changes in the structure of a part will alter the function, and the degree of change will be determined by the proportions it assumes. The divisions between normal and pathologic conditions are not always clearly delineated and thus create difficulties in making both diagnosis and prognosis. There is within the living animal characteristics that may allow adaptations without any noticeable effect, while others may manifest themselves and become acute. Recovery from each type of change is possible, but the possibility of death occurring is also present.

By applying the knowledge gained through the years, man is today experiencing a longer and healthier life. We are able to recognize diseases earlier and thus begin corrective treatments that contribute to increasing longevity. Preventive medicine is being practiced, thereby reducing the number of people contacting diseases who otherwise would require treatment. Many national and international organizations are addressing themselves to the task of personal hygiene and through this approach are experiencing successes that also perform a beneficial function in extending man's longevity. There are some diseases that have through the years extracted a high toll in human life but are today being treated successfully and even eliminated, only to have newer ones isolated or discovered that necessitate a continuous search for treatments and cures. X-rays have undoubtedly played an important role in the progress attained to date and have assisted scientific minds to understand in greater depth those diseases that in the past were known but not as completely or thoroughly understood as they are today. Much has been learned about the beneficial attributes of radiation and its value in diagnosing diseases, but we have also learned some of the deleterious effects that may occur and necessitate rigorous control and judicious application.

Anything that impairs normal function should in most instances be considered detrimental and consequently treated as such. All diseases may be subdivided into two categories or classifications: those that may be treated by medicine or therapeutic means, usually having a good prognosis, are termed medical diseases, while those requiring excision or removal to assure a good prognosis are termed surgical diseases. A listing of some of the diseases technologists should recognize and be familiar with, as well as their effects upon body functions, follow.

What is pathologic anatomy?

Pathologic anatomy is the study of structural changes.

What is a diagnosis?

In speaking about diagnosis we mean that a definite distinction has been made between one disease and another. A particular disease or condition has been recognized.

What is a prognosis?

When one is aware of the course of a particular disease, a prognosis, or forecast of the probable result of a disease, is made.

Define pathology.

Pathology is the science dealing with the cause and course of a disease. It is a study of the essential nature of diseases and especially of the structural and functional changes produced by them.

Define anomaly.

An anomaly is a malformation. Any organ or structure that is abnormal with respect to form, position, or structure is said to be an anomaly. Another definition would be "different from or contrary to the general rule."

To what does the term congenital refer?

It refers to formation prior to birth and present at birth, or inborn. Something said to be congenital was caused by changes taking place in the fetus during its developmental stages in the womb.

What is a congenital anomaly?

By combining the two previous definitions, we define it as "a malformation or abnormal form or position of a structure formed in the fetal stages and present at birth."

What is "osteogenesis imperfecta" and what is its effect?

Osteogenesis imperfecta is a disease involving the tissues developing from the primitive mesenchyme. It is a disorder of bone formation characterized by increased fragility of the bone. This fragility of bones results in an extremely large number of fractures caused by the very slightest possible trauma. The condition occurs at all ages but is seen chiefly in infants and has been diagnosed in utero.

How may one detect the condition of "osteopetrosis," or "marble bone"?

This condition, also known as Albers-

Schönberg disease, begins during fetal life and is characterized by obliteration of the medullary spaces, marked osseous density, and sclerosis. The bones are extremely brittle and will usually have multiple fractures. The fractures usually heal. The liver, spleen, and lymph nodes are enlarged.

What is sickle cell anemia?

Sickle cell anemia is a chronic hemolytic anemia characterized by dyspnea, pain in the abdomen and extremities, epistaxis, and the presence of sickle-shaped red blood cells. Cells affected in the sickling process become inflexible and fixed. They may increase in length, causing capillary blockage and resulting in stasis of blood in the capillaries and the small blood vessels, causing thrombosis and infarcts.

Define a pathologic fracture.

A pathologic fracture is a fracture occurring in a diseased bone. Such a fracture is dependent upon the underlying pathologic process. Pathologic changes may be local and restricted to one bone or segment of bone or may be systemic in origin and involve multiple bones or the entire skeleton.

What is the definition of "bolus" as regards anatomy and physiology?

The term "bolus" means a mass, a congregation of more tissue, for example, in a specific area than is otherwise normally present.

What is anoxia?

A condition produced by a deficiency in the supply of oxygen is known as anoxia. This condition may also appear as a respiratory obstruction caused by a reduced surface area in lungs for the exchange of gases or inadequate respiratory movements.

What is fibrosis?

Fibrosis means containing or composed of fibers. An abnormal amount of fibrous

tissue formation is observed in individuals who have had unusual numbers of pregnancies or those having had syphilis.

Define atrophy.

All structures grow or develop at a relativity normal rate until maturity. Once maturity has been reached and growth is functionally completed, any decrease in size will be referred to as atrophy. It may be simply defined as a reduction in size of any structure after it has reached full functional maturity.

What is osteoporosis and how may it be characterized?

Osteoporosis is an absorption of bone with the result that the tissue becomes unusually porous and fragile; it is characterized by a decrease in bone mass caused by a decrease in the production of osteoid by the osteoblasts. There is also a decrease in bone density resulting from interference with the process of matrix formation. This decalcification or loss of bone substance is important in making a diagnosis.

In examining a patient the clinician or diagnostician states that he has an objective sign. To what is he referring?

An objective sign is something that can be felt, seen, or heard by the examining clinician or diagnostician.

What is etiology?

Etiology is a derivative of the Greek word *aitiologia,* meaning cause. It is the study of the cause and origin of disease or abnormal conditions.

What does the word "coccus" mean?

Coccus is a spherical bacterium or a berry-shaped organism. It is one of the main groups of pathogenic bacteria.

Define briefly rheumatic fever.

Rheumatic fever is an acute, systemic

disease characterized by fever, inflammation, and pain and is variable in severity, duration, and sequelae. It is one of the leading diseases affecting the heart.

What causes cretinism or dwarfism?

Cretinism or dwarfism results from a deficiency or low output of hormones by the thyroid gland.

In what does a partial block of the renal artery usually result?

A partial block of the renal artery usually results in high blood pressure, or hypertension.

What is bronchiectasis?

Bronchiectasis is the dilation of a bronchus or bronchi on one or both sides of the chest. It usually results from obstructions and infections and usually is characterized by secretion of large amounts of offensive pus. It is important in causing lung abscess.

What is usually the cause of tumors of the secondary or metastatic type in the lungs?

Such tumors are caused by the extensions of the disease by passage through the bloodstream.

What is a carcinoma?

A carcinoma is a malignant neoplasm comprised of epithelial cells that tends to invade surrounding tissue and to metastasize by transfer of cells.

What is nephrolithiasis?

The prefix *nephro* relates to the kidney, and the term "nephrolithiasis" relates to the formation of calcified deposits or renal stones in the kidneys.

What are the three main groups of disease processes?

The three main groups are inflammation, degeneration, and tumefaction.

What is arteriosclerosis?

Arteriosclerosis is the term applied to pathologic conditions in which there is thickening, hardening, and loss of elasticity of the walls of blood vessels. This usually results in a disturbance of the blood flow to an organ.

Tuberculosis is an infectious disease caused by the tubercle bacillus. What areas of the body does it affect?

It commonly affects the respiratory system, but other parts may become infected. Other areas affected may be gastrointestinal and genitourinary systems, bones, joints, nervous system, lymph nodes, and skin.

What is a thrombus?

A thrombus is a blood clot that, when formed, may detach and progress with the bloodstream.

What is atelectasis?

The collapse of all or part of a lung is known as atelectasis.

What type of metastases causes a hole in bone?

Osteolytic.

What is osteomyelitis?

Osteomyelitis is an infectious inflammatory disease of bone marked by local death and separation of tissue.

What is empyema?

Empyema is the presence of pus in a body cavity. It also may be defined as a pleurisy with pus.

Where will a patient in shock show a rearrangement?

A rearrangement will be shown in the extracellular, intracellular, and intravascular fluid compartments.

What is caused by blocking arterial blood flow, the airway, or cellular respiration?

Anoxia, which can be of such severity to

cause or result in permanent damage, is caused by blockage.

What is a spirochete?

A spirochete is a spiral-shaped micro-organism.

A benign stricture or fibrous narrowing of the lower esophagus is caused by what?

The reflex of gastric secretions causes the stricture.

A blockage to the flow of biliary fluids is usually caused by what?

A carcinoma of the ampulla of Vater blocks the flow of biliary fluid.

What is cholecystitis?

Inflammation of the gallbladder is known as cholecystitis.

What causes gigantism?

Disease in the pituitary gland is a direct cause of gigantism.

The thyroid gland is frequently the site of what?

Goiters, which are usually visible as a swelling at the front of the neck, are often located in the thyroid gland.

Viruses are responsible for a variety of symptoms and conditions. What is the most well-known type of ailment attributed to viruses?

Pneumonia, which is a pneumococcus or respiratory disease, is the most well-known type of virus ailment.

What affects the production of the digestive enzymes?

Disease of the pancreas affects production.

The term "volvulus" refers to what?

Volvulus refers to a twisting of the bowel upon itself, causing obstruction.

What spreads malignant tumors?

The lymphatic system transports the disease to other areas of the body.

What is meant by stenosis?

Stenosis is a disease of the heart that results from valvular infection, which causes the cusps to become inflamed, and resultant fibrous tissue, which permanently narrows the valvular opening, thereby diminishing the flow of blood through it.

What is mitral stenosis?

Mitral stenosis is the infection of the mitral valve and is one of the most serious forms of heart disease. Blood flow from the left atrium into the left ventricle is markedly diminished so that there is a backflow into the lungs and the right side of the heart.

What is the importance of cardiac catheterization and angiocardiography in the study of heart disease?

Cardiac catheterization confirms the pressure and oxygen content of the heart chambers and great vessels. Angiocardiography provides radiographic visualization of the heart chambers, the aorta, and the pulmonary artery. Both of these together increase the accuracy of diagnostic procedures.

What is dyspnea?

Dyspnea is a condition of the heart caused by the interference with blood circulation; it is characterized by shortness of breath resulting from the inability of the heart to pump blood into the lungs for purification. The impure blood, upon reaching the brain, causes it to stimulate the respiratory center, thus making the patient breathe rapidly and have the feeling of shortness of breath.

What is atherosclerosis?

Atherosclerosis is a degenerative form of arteriosclerosis. It is a typically nodular thickening of the intima of the aorta and other arteries by lipids, with consequent reduction in the vessel's lumen and in the blood supply to the affected organs.

Localized dilatation of the artery is known as what?

This dilatation of the artery is known as an aneurysm. The dilatation may be fusiform, an elongate, spindle-shaped dilatation spread over the entire artery, or saccular, a saclike bulging of the artery at a particular point.

Emphysema is a disease of what anatomic part?

Emphysema is one of the serious pulmonary diseases and is characterized by the inability of the patient to breathe adequately. Its far-reaching effects are characterized by the barrel-shaped chest, diminished respiratory movements, and difficult and prolonged respiration of the patient.

What is pneumoconiosis?

Pneumoconiosis is an interstitial pneumonia caused by the irritation of the lungs by certain dust particles that are inhaled over an extended time period during employment in certain industrial processes.

The silica element in the dust is considered to be the most dangerous. Silicosis, the oldest and most serious of the diseases, is contracted by the inhalation of fine particles of silica over long periods of time in occupations such as gold mining, tin mining, stone working, metal grinding, or sand blasting.

Anthracosis is characteristic of the coal mining industry and is caused by the lungs becoming filled with coal dust.

Asbestosis is caused by the inhalation of asbestos dust by employees in that industry. The dust may be inhaled during the actual rock crushing procedure or in the manufacture of asbestos.

What is pleurisy?

Pleurisy is the inflammation of the pleura, a serous membrane enveloping the lungs and lining the walls of the thoracic cavity. It is characterized by the formation of a scratchy, inflammatory fibrin fluid, which covers the lung and chest wall pleura with a rough layer. When the patient breathes, the two rough layers come in contact with each other and in the act of rubbing together produce sharp pain in the side. The accumulation of fluid within the pleural cavity is known as pleurisy with effusion.

What is a pneumothorax?

Pneumothorax is air in the pleural cavity. Whatever the cause, whether it be internal or external in source, air accumulates in the pleural cavity, compressing the lung and causing a collapse.

In discussing diseases of the mouth, explain gingivitis and periodontitis.

Gingivitis is an inflammation of the gingiva, which is a mucous membrane surrounding the tooth. It is characterized by swollen and inflamed gums, with bleeding during the cleaning of teeth.

Periodontitis is a disease of the tooth's surrounding tissues in which a space appears between the root of a tooth and the bone.

What is dysentery?

Dysentery is an acute inflammation of the colon. It is a colitis characterized by acute diarrhea with liquid stools containing mucus, pus, and blood. There are two kinds of dysentery, amebic and bacillary.

What disease is coincidental with the vermiform appendix?

Appendicitis, caused by infection and obstruction is coincidental with the vermiform appendix.

The peritoneum is a serous membrane lining the walls of the abdominal cavity. It is

moistened with a lubricant reducing friction between surfaces. What is inflammation of this membrane called?

Inflammation of the peritoneum is called peritonitis. The inflammation is caused by infection generated by one of the organs covered by the membrane. Infection may be carried by the bloodstream. Peritonitis may be of two types, local or general. Local peritonitis is that which is limited to one area, for example, the appendix. General peritonitis is caused by the spreading of infection throughout the peritoneal cavity. Acute intestinal obstruction is one danger of general peritonitis.

What is a diverticulum and what disease is associated with it?

A diverticulum is the herniation, or bubbling out, of the mucosa at some point of weakness. Infection or inflammation occurring in the diverticula produces symptoms similar to those of appendicitis, except that they are left-sided.

Why is it important for children to receive accurate diagnosis and treatment of intussusception?

Intussusception is a cause of acute intestinal obstruction in children. Intussusception is the enfolding of one segment of the intestines into itself. The entering piece of intestine is quickly enfolded by the rest of the intestine and passed along by the peristaltic waves. The danger of intussusception is strangulation. The infolded piece of intestine is held captive and squeezed so tightly that the venous blood cannot return, thus causing swelling of the part. Arteries become compressed, the blood supply stops, and gangrene sets in. The resultant danger is acute abdominal obstruction and general peritonitis.

What is intestinal obstruction?

When material in the intestines is unable to be passed along its length, the con-

dition may be termed intestinal obstruction. There are two types of intestinal obstructions. They are organic and paralytic. Organic may be the result of blockage by some obstacle, such as a tumor or intestinal twisting. Paralytic obstruction results from a bowel segment inflammation, causing the stoppage of peristaltic movements from one section of bowel to the one immediately below. If peristaltic movements are unable to be passed along the length of the bowel, movement of the bowel ceases.

What is the function of insulin?

Insulin regulates carbohydrate metabolism. Production of insufficient insulin produces diabetes.

What is meant by diabetes?

The word "diabetes" simply means "to go through." However, when combined with the word "mellitus," which means sweet, indicating the presence of sugar, it indicates a pathologic condition of the pancreas that decreases the amount of insulin formed, therefore resulting in impaired carbohydrate metabolism and increased concentration of glucose in the blood and urine.

Injury to the posterior lobe of the pituitary may lead to an antidiuretic hormonal deficiency, causing diabetes insipidus. This hormonal deficiency leads to the nonconcentration of urine in the kidneys, thus allowing the output of a patient's urine to reach 30 or 40 liters per day instead of the normal 1.2 to 1.5 liters. In addition, the patient suffers from excessive thirst.

What is meant by hypertension?

Hypertension is defined as high blood pressure.

Pyelonephritis is associated with what organ of the body?

Pyelonephritis is associated with the kidney and means inflammation of the kidney and renal pelves. The inflammation is primarily an inflammation of the interstitial tissue rather than the parenchyma of the kidney.

Nutritional deficiency, combined with alcohol, is a common factor producing what disease?

Nutritional deficiency, combined with large continuous intake of alcohol, is a common factor producing cirrhosis of the liver. Damage to the liver resulting from viral, toxic, or deficiency hepatitis provides a progressive chronic destruction of the organ.

How can jaundice be recognized by the technologist?

Jaundice can be noted by the technologist in remembering that in certain impairments of the functioning of the liver bile pigments accumulate in the blood and tissues, giving a yellowish tinge to the skin and whites of the eyes. The color may vary from pale yellow to a deep orange.

Jaundice occurs when the normally functioning liver excretes bile, but because of a stoppage in the hepatic or common bile ducts the bile is not allowed to enter the duodenum. The bile is pooled within the ductile system and eventually backs up into the liver, where the bile enters the blood. This condition is known as obstructive jaundice.

Hepatitis creates a condition in which the liver becomes unable to excrete the bilirubin, and since there is no other method of excretion, the bilirubin is absorbed into the blood. This disease is hepatic jaundice.

An intravenous pyelogram examination is ordered to determine the presence of urinary calculus. What does this mean?

The request for an intravenous pyelogram suggests the presence of a urinary calculus, or stone, that forms in the urinary tract. Kidney stones form in the kidneys, but some stones may have their origin in the bladder. The renal pelvis becomes the originator of the kidney stone and from this the stone passes into the bladder by means of the ureter. Bladder stones may have their origination within the bladder but most often are the result of kidney stones passing down from above. The causes for the formation of stones are problematic, but the following may be considered: infection, high concentration of crystalline salts in the urine, vitamin-poor diet, and tumors of the parathyroid glands.

Dilatation of the renal pelvis caused by urine accumulation is indicative of what disease?

When a kidney stone becomes lodged in the ureter, stopping the passage of urine into the bladder, the result is an accumulation of urine causing a dilatation of the renal pelvis. This condition is known as hydronephrosis.

What is anuria?

A patient who has anuria has a condition in which the kidneys do not excrete urine.

What is meant by the diagnosis of uremia?

If the kidneys do not excrete, there is an accumulation of poisonous waste products in the bloodstream and in our body tissues. This condition is known as uremia.

What is hyperthyroidism?

Hyperthyroidism is a disease consistent with the overactivity of the thyroid gland, with extreme amounts of thyroxin produced.

What is the chief value of blood transfusions?

The chief value of blood transfusions is the replacement of blood lost after acute hemorrhaging. It is useful to alleviate shock following loss of blood in traumas and in surgical operations.

What is anemia?

Anemia is not a single, specific disease but rather a condition that has many causes. It is characterized by a decrease in the number of red cells in the blood, by a decrease in the amount of hemoglobin per red cell, or by both. There is a marked drop in the number of red cells per cubic millimeter of blood.

What is polycythemia?

The term "polycythemia" means an increase in the number of circulating red cells per cubic millimeter. True polycythemia results from an overproduction of red cells. The blood becomes very viscous and tends to plug the blood vessels.

What do you understand the disease hemophilia to be?

The hereditary disease hemophilia, a sex-linked trait transmitted from generation to generation, is characterized by such defective clotting of the blood that a slight scratch may lead to a fatal hemorrhage. The disease affects males primarily and is transmitted to them from their mothers.

What is leukemia?

Leukemia is a disease of the cells that produce white corpuscles. It is important to realize that leukemia is essentially a cancer of the bone marrow and not of the blood.

What disease is characterized by an increase in the number of white blood cells above the normal?

Leukocytosis is characterized by an increase in the number of white cells above the normal.

What is the oldest of all known diseases?

The oldest of all known diseases is the common crippling disease known as chronic arthritis. This is a chronic inflammatory condition affecting small joints of the hands and feet, although larger joints may be affected later. Rheumatoid arthritis is one of the largest causes of disability in the United States.

What causes degeneration of articular cartilage and bone?

Osteoarthritis is the degeneration of articular cartilage and bone caused by an inflammation of the synovial membrane. It is usually called a degenerative arthritis, and it affects both men and women in later periods of life.

What is a "slipped disk"?

A slipped disk is a condition in which the intervertebral disk has either become protruded or herniated into the vertebral canal and presses on the spinal cord or stretches the nerve. This condition occurs at the sites of maximum anterior spinal curvature, usually between the region of the fourth lumbar and first sacral spine or between the fifth and seventh cervical vertebrae.

What is necrosis?

Necrosis is the death of cells. The death of the cells may result from chemical poisons, bacterial toxins, irradiation, or other physical agents, or loss of blood supply from arterial closure.

What functions do the body systems perform?

The circulatory system is a mechanism that sends fresh material (food and oxygen) to the tissue fluid and removes waste material from it.

The respiratory system is designed to bring oxygen from outside the body to the innermost portions.

The digestive system is concerned with the breakdown and preparation of the food that is fed to the tissues of the body by the bloodstream.

The excretory system functions as the waste remover of the body. The nervous system acts as the message center for the body, controlling all messages to the various portions of the body.

The reproductive system, perhaps the most complex of all mechanisms of the body, has the function of reproducing the organism.

What is pathogenesis?

Pathogenesis is defined as the method of production and development of the lesion, while the causation of a pathologic process is known as etiology.

Define trauma, fracture, and wound.

Trauma is an injury causing damage to a particular portion of the body to the extent that tissues may be killed. It may be a sharp blow, a wound, a bone fracture, or even a sprain to one of the joints. Lesser degrees of trauma may cause inflammation.

Fracture may be defined as a breaking of the bone. Simple fracture is that in which a bone is broken but the broken ends do not penetrate the skin. A compound fracture is one in which the broken ends of the bone are projected through the skin. A greenstick fracture, usually found in children, is characterized by the cracking of the bone, although it is not completely shattered. Since the bones of a child are soft and pliable, the fracture resembles the bending of a green twig.

A wound is an injury in which the skin has been broken.

What is the most common cause of disease?

The most common cause of disease known to man is bacteria. Molds or fungi belong in the vegetable kingdom, but it should be remembered that animal parasites may inhabit the body and produce disease.

What is ischemia?

Ischemia is the loss of blood supply to a local area or part.

What is the cause of vitamin deficiency?

Vitamin deficiency may be caused by the inadequate intake of food, or the food taken in, although adequate, may not be used properly.

What are the five major vitamin deficiency diseases?

The five major vitamin deficiency diseases are beriberi—vitamin B complex, thiamine; pellagra—vitamin B complex, niacin; scurvy—vitamin C; rickets—vitamin D; keratomalacia—vitamin A.

What is rickets?

Rickets is a disease of young children characterized by improperly formed bones caused by the insufficient deposition of both calcium and phosphorus. The bones are soft and bend easily, causing deformities. It may be caused by one or both of the following: insufficient vitamin D or insufficient sunlight.

What diseases are associated with the following vitamin deficiencies: vitamin A, thiamine (B_1), riboflavin (B_2), niacin (B_{12}), vitamin C, vitamin D, vitamin K?

Vitamin A deficiency causes night blindness. Thiamine (B_1) deficiency results in beriberi. Riboflavin (B_2) deficiency contributes to eye lesions. Niacin deficiency causes pellagra. Vitamin B_{12} deficiency causes pernicious anemia; vitamin C deficiency, scurvy; vitamin D deficiency, rickets; and vitamin K, when deficient, causes a tendency to bleeding.

Laboratory examinations are an integral part of diagnosis. They are numerous and complex. Of what value are the following laboratory procedures in assisting diagnosis: urinalysis, blood count, bacteriologic examination, serology, tissue diagnosis, basal metabolism?

Urinalysis, the most common of all laboratory examinations, provides for the examination of the urine to indicate conditions of the kidneys and reveal diseases of the bladder and urethra. A urinalysis will show the presence of sugar in the urine to indicate diabetes.

The blood count shows the number and conditions of red blood cells and leukocytes. In anemia the red cells are diminished and can be counted. Acute infections will produce an increase in the leukocytes.

Bacteriologic examination assists in the diagnosis of infectious diseases. A blood culture shows the presence of streptococci and other organisms in the circulating blood.

Serology, while a branch of bacteriology, examines the blood serum for substances that indicate the presence of bacterial infection.

Tissue diagnosis is the microscopic examination of tissue pieces.

Basal metabolism is the determination of the heat production of the body. It is determined by the amount of oxygen consumed over a given period of time.

What is an embolus?

An embolus is a clot that has detached itself from the circulatory system wall and has entered the bloodstream as a freely floating object. The clot may start in a vein and proceed through the circulatory system to the heart. As it approaches the heart, it meets little resistance as the veins become larger. It is usually after the thrombus passes through the heart that trouble begins, because of the narrowing of the smaller arteries.

What is edema?

Edema is the abnormal local or generalized collection of fluid in the tissue spaces.

What is the appearance of a person in shock?

The symptoms of a person in shock are invariable. The patient's face is very pale, and the skin is cold and clammy. The temperature is subnormal, with the pulse feeble. Blood pressure remains relatively low, and the patient's breathing is shallow, with occasional sighing.

REFERENCE

Potsaid, M. (Director of Radiological Research and Development, and Director of Nuclear Medicine, Massachusetts General Hospital): Personal communication.

6 ANATOMY AND PHYSIOLOGY

What is anatomy?

Anatomy is the science dealing with the structure of the body and the relationship of its parts.

What constitutes the structure?

The structure is the skeleton or bony framework that gives shape and form to the body. It protects vital organs and provides places of attachment for ligaments, muscles, and tendons.

What is physiology?

Physiology is the study of the functions of the organs of the body.

What is tissue?

A tissue may be defined as a group or layer of similarly specialized cells that together perform certain special functions. Histology is the study of the structure and arrangement of tissues. Each kind of tissue is composed of cells that have a characteristic size, shape, and arrangement. Tissues may consist of matter other than living cells. Some nonliving material is contained between the cells of blood and the connective tissues.

Describe briefly the classifications of tissues.

While there is some difference of opinion as to the classification of tissues, we shall restrict the description to four types of tissue, namely, epithelial, connective, muscular, and nervous.

Epithelial tissues are composed of cells that form a continuous layer or sheet covering the body surface or lining body cavities. Their functions concern protection, absorption, secretion, and sensation.

Connective tissue supports and holds together other cells of the body. Examples of connective tissues are bones, cartilages, tendons, ligaments, and fibrous connective tissues. Matrix, a nonliving material, is secreted by the cells of the connective tissues. This secretion becomes the bonding and supporting material between the cells.

Muscular tissue controls the contractions of muscles. The tissues are composed of elongated cylindrical or spindle-shaped cells, each of which contains many small, longitudinal parallel contractile fibers. Three types of muscle are found in the human body. They are skeletal, smooth, and cardiac.

Nervous tissue functions in the conduction of electrochemical nerve impulses. Nerve fibers, composed of cytoplasm and protected by a plasma membrane, vary in size. The neuron cells join together to pass impulses over long distances throughout the body.

What is mitosis?

A property of living matter is its ability to renew or increase itself. This renewal or increase in the growth of a tissue is the result of a multiplication of cell members resulting from the division of the protoplasm, which is preceded by the division of its nucleus. The regularity of the process of cell division ensures that each cell will receive exactly the same number and kind of chromosomes that the parent cell had. Mitosis, then, is the regular division of a cell in such a fashion that each of the two resultant cells receives exactly the same number and the same kind of chromosomes that the parent cell had. The cellular division involves longitudinal (lengthwise) splitting of the chromosomes so that they form identical halves.

Describe cell structure.

Protoplasm forms the mass of the cell. It is gelatinous and semifluid and is thought to consist of a mobile framework of protein molecules along with fatty materials, carbohydrates, and salts. The outer surface of each cell is bounded by a delicate, elastic covering called the plasma membrane. This membrane regulates the contents of the cell, for all nutrients entering the cell and all waste products or secretions leaving the cell must pass through it.

The nucleus is a small spherical or oval body, usually found near the center in a relatively fixed position. However, it may move around and be found almost anywhere within the cell. It appears to consist of a clear fluid in which are strands supporting dense granules contained in a nuclear membrane. The granules are known as chromatin. The nucleus directs many aspects of cellular activity and contains the hereditary factors (genes) responsible for the traits of the organism.

The nuclear membrane surrounds the nucleus and separates it from the rest of the cell, regulating the flow of materials in and out of the nucleus.

Cytoplasm is a semifluid material within the plasma membrane, yet outside the nucleus. In this semifluid are found droplets, vacuoles, granules, and fibrils.

Centrioles are small cylindrical bodies adjacent to the nucleus that play a prominent role at the time of cell division. Endoplasmic reticulum (processes) are tubular strand membranes resembling small spaghetti spreading out from the cytoplasm of the cell.

What is meant by an organ?

An organ is a single unit of a system that is composed of various types of tissues that together perform a particular function. Examples of organs are the heart, liver, kidneys, and lungs.

Define and describe the various systems in the body.

A system is a group of organs composed of several types of tissues in which a division of labor has occurred and in which each performs some part of the principal life functions.

In man we can find the following systems:

1. The circulatory system transports materials throughout the body.
2. The respiratory system provides the exchange of oxygen and carbon dioxide.
3. The digestive system provides for the food intake, breakdown and absorption of food.
4. The excretory system is concerned with the elimination of waste products from the body.
5. The skeletal system provides for locomotion and support of the body.
6. The muscular system provides for movement and locomotion in conjunction with the skeletal system.
7. The nervous system conducts impulses around the body and integrates the activities of other systems.

8. The endocrine system serves as a coordinator of body functions.
9. The reproductive system deals with the continuation of the species.
10. The sensory system receives stimuli from outside and from within the body.

What factors determine the density of tissue and organs?

The density of the various organs within the body system will vary considerably in the radiographic process and will depend upon the composition of cellular structure, the intracellular space-taking fluid, and the anatomic makeup of the organ itself—whether it is solid, empty, or filled with some material.

What function does the skin serve?

The most obvious of its functions are that of protection of the body against outside environmental bacteria and help in maintaining a constant internal environment. It shields the underlying cells from injuries caused by blows, friction, or pressure.

If the skin remains unbroken, it is relatively germproof, and protection is afforded the body against disease-producing organisms.

The waterproof quality of the skin protects the body from excessive loss of moisture.

The skin protects the underlying cells from the harmful ultraviolet rays of the sun by virtue of the pigment it can produce (suntan).

The skin functions as a thermostat, controlling the elimination of heat from the body and insulating it from the cold.

The skin functions as an excretory system through the elimination of secretions via the sweat glands of the skin.

The skin contains a number of sense receptors responsible for our ability to feel pressure, temperature changes, and pain.

It also enables us to discriminate between the various objects that are touched.

Describe the structure of bone.

The periosteum is a vascular membrane having many blood vessels at the end and covering the bone. It is a tough, fibrous, highly sensitive membrane, with the outer layer more vascular and the inner layer lined in the growing bone; it contains bone-forming cells called osteoblasts. Deposits of bone from the inner layer upon the surface of the shaft provide for growth of bone in thickness and assist in the repair of broken bones.

Lying under the periosteum is the cortex, which is composed of dense, compact bone. The thickness of the cortical layer in the bones will vary with the classification of bones. For example, there will be a thick layer of compact bone in the shaft of the long bones, while in the flat and irregular bones the layer is thin.

Cancellous bone is the inner spongy, porous section forming a layer under the cortex.

The cavity of the shaft of the bone is called the medulla, and the lining of the bone cavity is called endosteum.

Bone marrow is the tissue contained within the cavity of the long bones. Yellow bone marrow is found chiefly in the adult and is made up primarily of fat. The red marrow contains little fat but is supplied with blood and reddish-colored cells called erythroblasts, from which red blood cells are formed.

Nutrient foramina are small openings that extend down through each bone and contain one or more blood vessels to the bone.

The supply of blood to the bone is received through one large nutrient artery tunneling the bone obliquely to gain the marrow cavity. It divides into two branches, one for each end for the marrow and spongy bone.

How are bones classified?

Bones are classified as long, short, flat, and irregular. Long bones have two extremities and a shaft. They are provided with a medullary canal, which contains marrow. The femur is an example of a long bone.

Short bones are small and irregular in shape. They are made of cancellous tissue, except for a thin layer of compact tissue covering the surface. The bones of the wrist and ankle are examples of short bones.

Flat bones afford extensive protection and broad surfaces for the attachment of muscles. The skull bones, sternum, and scapula are examples of flat bones.

Irregular bones are those that cannot be placed in any other category because of their peculiar shape. A vertebra is an example of an irregular bone.

Explain the meaning of the following: diaphysis, epiphysis, epiphyseal line, and metaphysis.

Diaphysis is the bone formed from the primary center of ossification in the shaft. The growth in the length of the bone is for the most part the result of the growth of cartilage followed by the deposition of bone to the shaft along the line of the epiphyseal plate.

The epiphysis is a term employed to denote the extremities of long bones. The epiphysis is formed by the secondary centers of ossification.

The epiphyseal line is a thin plate of cartilage separating the diaphysis from the epiphysis and is vitally important in the longitudinal growth of the bone. As the diaphysis grows, the epiphysis enlarges by the activity of its cartilage cells to keep its place. The deep layer of its articular cartilage is replaced by bone. The cells of the cartilage keep multiplying in front of the advancing bone until nature decides that the growth requisite for the individual has been reached. The epiphysis then fuses to the shaft.

The metaphysis is the part of the diaphysis that is the end of the shaft next to the epiphysis.

How are the joints of the body classified?

The joints of the body are classified into three main divisions.

Immovable joints, or fibrous joints, are so called because fibrous tissues unite the joint, limiting the motion. In the syndesmosis variety, the bones are a short distance apart but held firmly by interosseous ligaments that permit little movement. The suture, with a thin layer of fibrous tissue, permits no movement and usually becomes ossified in later life. It is found in the skull.

Slightly movable joints, or cartilaginous joints, are found where cartilage unites the bones. This is demonstrated where the bones are coated with hard hyaline cartilage and united by disks of softer fibrocartilage. These joints grant limited motion, as seen between the vertebral bodies.

In the freely movable joints, or synovial joints, the bones move easily upon each other because they are plated with smooth articular cartilage, kept oiled by the synovial fluid.

Name and explain the various types of freely moving joints.

The gliding joint is a sliding of one surface over another without angular or rotary movement. Wherever two bones move one on another, their ends do not touch directly but are covered with smooth, slippery cartilage that reduces friction. Examples of the gliding joint are the intercarpal bones of the wrist, the intertarsal bones of the foot, and the vertebrae.

The hinge joint occurs with angular movement, as seen in the bending of the elbow and knee. When bending the elbow, the angle is decreased and we note that the elbow is in flexion; when the elbow is straightened and the angle is increased, we use the term "extension."

A saddle joint occurs with two angular movements at right angles to each other, back and forth and side to side. An example of this type of joint occurs at the carpometacarpal joint of the thumb.

A pivot joint affords rotational movement of the bone around its own longitudinal axis. A typical pivot joint is seen in the pivoting of the radius, rotating in the ring formed by the ulna and the annular ligament.

The ball and socket joint is best typified by the hip joint and the shoulder joint, where the rounded head of a bone fits into a concave cavity of another bone.

The condyloid joint is described as having circumduction, which is a combination of the movements of flexion, abduction, extension, and adduction. The metacarpophalangeal joints of the fingers are condyloid joints.

What is meant by the terms "axial skeleton" and "appendicular skeleton"?

The axial skeleton includes the skull, vertebrae, ribs, and sternum. The skull is made up of a number of bones fused together. The vertebrae, or spine, are thirty-three separate vertebral bones that differ in size and shape at different points along the spine. The various vertebral bodies have different projections for the attachment of ribs and muscles and for articulating with other vertebral bodies above and below. The rib cage is composed of a series of flat bones attached dorsally to the vertebrae. Each pair of ribs is attached to a separate vertebra. The first seven pairs of ribs are anteriorly attached to the sternum. The eighth, ninth, and tenth pairs of ribs are attached indirectly to the sternum by cartilage. The eleventh and twelfth pairs are not attached to the sternum.

The appendicular skeleton is composed of the upper and lower extremities, the pelvis, and the shoulder girdles. The bones of the upper extremity are the humerus (upper arm), the radius and ulna (lower arm), the carpal bones of the wrist, the metacarpals of the hand, and the phalanges or fingers. The upper extremity is attached to the body by means of the shoulder girdle, which consists of a clavicle, or collar bone, and a scapula, or shoulder blade. The shoulder girdle is attached to the body by means of muscles.

The lower extremity bones are the femur (thigh), the fibula and tibia (lower leg), the tarsal bones, the metatarsal bones, and the phalanges of the toes. The patella (kneecap) is a separate bone in the lower extremity. The lower extremity is attached to the body by means of the pelvic girdle, which consists of three fused bones. Unlike the shoulder girdle, the pelvic girdle is fused to the vertebral column.

What functions do the muscles perform?

Muscles perform the actions of contraction and movement. Muscles do not contract as individuals but always in group action. For example, contracting the biceps muscle without bending the elbow would not be possible. One must remember that muscles do not exert pushing action, only pulling. Therefore, one can usually find muscles in pairs, pulling in opposite directions to each other. When one muscle contracts, the opposing muscle must relax to permit movement.

Muscles are used to maintain posture in the stopped position. In this position there is little activity necessary in the abdominal, thigh, or anterior leg muscles, but the calf muscles are active.

When muscles are not contracting to effect a movement, they are not completely relaxed. As long as a person is conscious, all muscles are contracted slightly. This condition gives support to the joints and is useful in promoting quick movement when needed.

What is meant by muscle tonus?

A muscle fully relaxed may contract to approximately half its length but retain its full state of tension. This condition is known as muscle tonus.

What is systolic and diastolic pressure?

Blood pressure increases with increased force of the heart beat and blood volume and the constriction of blood vessels. Just the opposite forces decrease pressure. The pressure rises with each contraction and falls with each relaxation of the ventricles. The highest pressure, caused by the contraction of the heart, is called systolic pressure. The lowest pressure, resulting from the relaxing of the heart, is called diastolic pressure.

If a patient were to faint in the x-ray department, where would you, as a technologist, expediently attempt to ascertain the condition of pulse?

While there are several anatomic landmarks for securing the pulse, the following would probably be the most expedient for the technologist in attempting to find the pulse.
1. The radial artery may be found laterally on the anterior surface of the wrist.
2. The ulnar artery may be found medially and on the anterior surface of the wrist.
3. The superficial temporal may be found directly anterior to the external auditory meatus.
4. The femoral artery may be found in the groin.

What is metabolism?

Metabolism is the sum of all the chemical activities of the cell that provide for its growth, maintenance, and repair. All cells constantly change by taking in new materials, altering them chemically in a variety of ways, and building new cellular material. The transformation of potential energy contained in the large molecules of carbohydrates, fats, and proteins is made through kinetic energy and heat as these

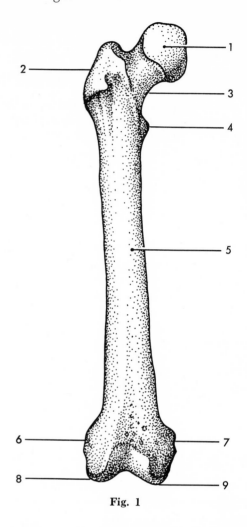

Fig. 1

substances are converted into other substances.

What are endocrine glands?

Endocrine, or ductless, glands are glands that are known to secrete substances into the bloodstream rather than into a duct leading to the outside of the body or to one of the other internal organs inside the body.

Name the endocrine glands.

The endocrine glands are as follows: pineal gland, pituitary gland, thyroid gland, parathyroid gland, thymus gland, the liver,

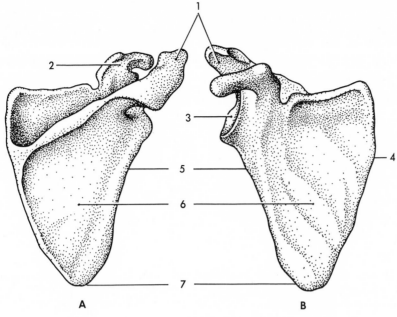

A   B

Fig. 2

the stomach, the duodenum, the pancreas, the adrenal gland, and the ovaries and testes.

Name the bone shown in Fig. 1 and list its parts.

The bone is the femur.
Parts:
1. Head
2. Greater trochanter
3. Neck
4. Lesser trochanter
5. Shaft
6. Lateral epicondyle
7. Medial epicondyle
8. Lateral condyle
9. Medial condyle

Name the bone shown in Fig. 2, identify the views, and name the parts.

The bone is the scapula. The views are posterior (*A*) and anterior (*B*).
Parts:
1. Acromion
2. Coracoid process

3. Glenoid cavity
4. Vertebral body
5. Axillary border
6. Inferior angle

Name the bones shown in Fig. 3.

1. Distal phalanx
2. Proximal phalanx
3. Sesamoid bone
4. Fifth metacarpal bone
5. Hamate bone
6. Pisiform bone
7. Triangular bone
8. Lunate bone
9. Greater multangular
10. Lesser multangular
11. Capitate bone
12. Navicular
13. Radius
14. Ulna

Name the parts of the pelvis shown in Fig. 4.

1. Sacrum
2. Sacroiliac joint

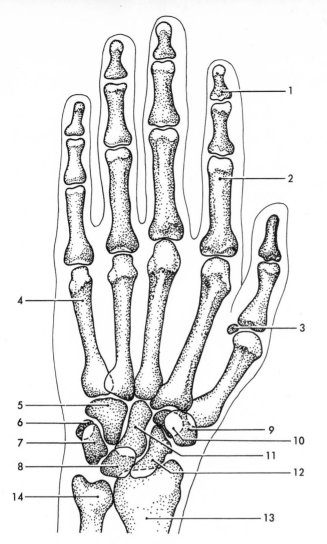

Fig. 3

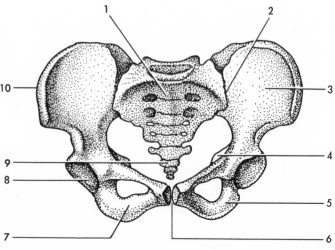

Fig. 4

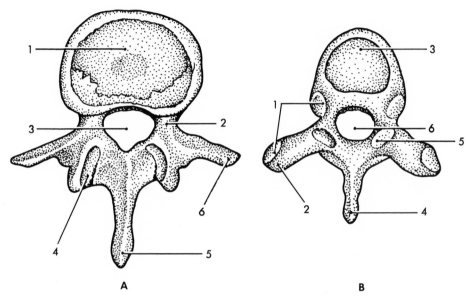

A   B

Fig. 5

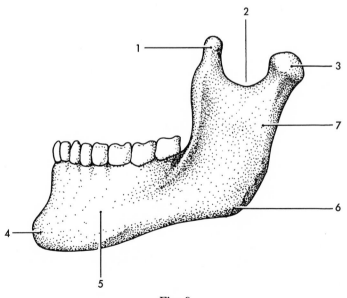

Fig. 6

3. Ilium
4. Ischium spine
5. Ischium
6. Symphysis pubis
7. Pubic bone
8. Acetabulum
9. Coccyx
10. Crest of ilium

Name the spines shown in Fig. 5 and list their parts.

The spines are lumbar (*A*) and thoracic (*B*).

A
1. Body
2. Pedicle
3. Vertebral foramen
4. Superior articular processes
5. Spinous process
6. Transverse process

B
1. Facet for rib
2. Transverse process
3. Body
4. Spinous process
5. Superior articular process
6. Vertebral foramen

Name the parts of the mandible as shown in Fig. 6.

1. Coronoid process
2. Mandibular notch
3. Capitulum
4. Mental protuberance
5. Angle of mandible
6. Ramus

What is the purpose of joints?

Joints permit movements, which are the results of the actions of muscles.

What kinds of movements are there? Define them.

pronation turning downward, such as the palm of the hand
supination turning upward, such as the palm of the hand
abduction moving away from the midline of the body

adduction moving toward the midline of the body
flexion bending, such as the elbow
extension straightening, such as the elbow
rotation turning on its axis, such as the head on the neck
inversion turning inward, such as the medial aspect of the foot
eversion turning outward, such as the lateral aspect of the foot

Parts of the body are referred to as being lateral, medial, inferior, or superior. Explain.

When a part is lateral, it is to the side; medial means toward the middle; inferior means below the midline, and superior means above it.

When we state that something is anterior or posterior, to what do we refer?

Anterior means to the front of the midline of the body, and posterior means to the back, or behind, the midline. If an imaginary line were drawn through the middle of a person, dividing the body into equal right and left halves, and again from the side, dividing into equal halves front and back, these divisions would then be classified as medial, lateral, anterior, and posterior, respectively, from the point of division.

Into how many parts is the skull divided?

The skull is divided into two parts, the cranium and the facial bones.

How many bones comprise the cranium, and what are they?

The cranium is made up of eight flat bones, united by sutures. They are the occipital bone, 1; temporal bones, 2; parietal bones, 2; sphenoid bone, 1; frontal bone, 1; and ethmoid bone, 1.

Describe the relationship of the bones of the cranium.

The occipital bone is located at the back and base of the skull. It forms and contains the foramen magnum. The temporal bones are on either side of the cranium, forming a portion of the lateral walls and the base of the skull. The parietal bones form most of the lateral and upper walls of the cranium. They articulate with each other at the midline, with the occipital posteriorly and the frontal anteriorly. The sphenoid bone lies in the anterior part of the base of the skull and articulates with the other seven bones of the cranium. The frontal bone forms the forehead and enters into the formation of the roof of the orbits and nasal cavities. The ethmoid bone lies in the anterior portion of the cranium. It forms part of the orbits, nasal fossa, and base of the cranium.

How many planes are in the skull? What are they?

There are four planes in the skull. They are the midsagittal, which divides the skull into right and left halves; vertical, which passes between the external auditory meatuses and is perpendicular to the horizontal plane; horizontal, which passes through the inferior margin of both orbits and the superior margin of both auditory meatuses; and the occlusal, which is an imaginary surface between the upper and lower teeth.

It has been stated previously that the bases of the cranium are joined by sutures. How many are there, and what are their names?

The bones of the cranium are joined by the following four sutures:

sagittal joins the two parietal bones at the top of the skull

coronal unites the frontal with the parietals and joins the sagittal

lambdoid unites the occipital and parietal

squamosal unites the temporal and parietal bones

The bones of the face are paired, with the exception of two. What two bones are these?

These two bones are the vomar and the mandible.

Name the three facial cavities.

The three facial cavities are as follows:

orbital pertaining to the eyes

nasal pertaining to the nose

oral pertaining to the mouth

Name and define the various areas within the skull called sinuses.

The bony cavities within the cranium and facial bones bearing the name of the associated bones are called sinuses. The sinuses add resonance to the voice.

maxillary sinuses within the superior maxilla

frontal sinuses within the frontal bone

ethmoid sinuses within the ethmoid bone

sphenoid sinuses within the sphenoid bone

Name the vertebrae of the body.

The body is composed of five sets of vertebrae. They are the cervical, dorsal, lumbar, sacral, and coccygeal.

How many vertebrae are there in each set?

The cervical vertebrae are seven in number; dorsal are twelve; lumbar are five; sacrum is composed of five vertebrae fused together and therefore classified as one bone; coccyx has four segments, which are also fused together.

How many parts are there to a vertebra? Name them.

There are seven parts of a vertebra. They are the body, neural arch, vertebral foramen, spinous process, transverse process, articular processes, lamina, pedicles, and transverse foramina.

Are the vertebrae of standard size and shape throughout?

No, they are not. The cervical vertebrae are smaller than the other vertebrae. They increase in size from the top downward, with each of the different sets of vertebrae being larger until reaching the sacrum.

What are the axis and atlas?

The axis is the second cervical vertebra and has on its superior surface a long, bony prominence called the odontoid, which fits into the opening of the atlas, or first cervical vertebra. (The atlas is the strongest of the cervical vertebrae.) The spinous process of the axis is very thick when compared to those of the other cervical vertebrae.

What is the difference between the thoracic vertebrae and the cervical and lumbar vertebrae?

The thoracic vertebrae have a distinctive characteristic in that they have facets on their sides for articulation with the heads of ribs. The other vertebrae do not have these facets since they do not articulate with ribs.

Do all thoracic vertebrae have facets and articulate with ribs?

Yes. The first eight vertebral bodies articulate with two pairs of ribs, the pair with which they correspond numerically and the pair below. The bodies of the lower four articulate with the pair of ribs with which they correspond numerically.

Describe the lumbar vertebrae.

The total lumbar vertebrae are five and are numbered from the top down. No bony articulations are present, except those for articulation with other vertebrae. They are larger than the cervical and most of the thoracic vertebrae. The bodies are larger, and the vertebral foramina are triangular in outline, with rounded corners. The spinous processes are large and hatchet shaped.

What type of joint is the articular processes of the vertebrae?

The joint separation between vertebrae is a gliding joint. There are disks of cartilage in the joint cavities. The bones are held together by ligaments, which are composed of tough, fibrous tissue.

Describe the sacrum.

The sacrum has the form of an inverted triangle and is composed of five sacral vertebrae fused together to increase the stability of the pelvis. It is located between the two hip bones and forms the greater part of the posterior wall of the pelvic cavity.

What is the coccyx?

The coccyx is the lowest or most inferior portion of the spinal column. It is usually made up of four segments, which may be fused together. It is triangular in outline with the apex below, with a curvature that is downward and forward.

For the purpose of describing the abdomen, it is divided into how many regions? What are they?

The abdomen is divided into nine regions by two horizontal and two vertical lines. The upper horizontal line passes through the tenth costal cartilage inferiorly, with the lower horizontal line passing through the level of the anterior superior iliac spine. The vertical lines pass through a point midway in the length of the inguinal ligament.

The regions above the upper horizontal line are the right and left hypochondriac and the epigastric. Between the horizontal lines are located the right and left lumbar and umbilical regions. Below the lower horizontal line are the right and left iliac and hypogastric regions.

Muscles are an important part of the physical structure of man, having a direct effect on movements. How many types of muscles are there, and what are their names?

There are three distinct types of muscles within the body. They are smooth muscles, which function involuntarily, that is, do not rely on stimuli from the brain to act; striated muscles, which function under control of the mind and comprise the skeletal muscles; and cardiac muscles, which are composed of cells that constitute the dynamic musculature of the heart. Cardiac muscles resemble both smooth and striated muscles.

What bones comprise the upper extremity?

The upper extremity is composed of the humerus, radius and ulna, clavicle, scapula, carpals, metacarpals, and phalanges. The total number of bones in the upper extremity is thirty-two.

The following terms are used in connection with the upper extremities. Describe each term listed below as it refers to the humerus: anatomic neck, radial fossa, olecranon fossa, shaft or body, greater tuberosity, surgical neck, and head.

anatomic neck that portion of the humerus located between the greater and lesser tuberosities of the head

radial fossa slight depression on the anterior aspect of the humerus, superior to the capitulum, for accepting the head of the radius during flexion of the forearm

olecranon fossa deep depression superior to the posterior aspect of the trochlea, which is the medial portion of the articular surface on the distal end of the humerus

shaft or body long portion of bone extending from the neck to the condyles, containing a central or medullary cavity

greater tuberosity large elevation (eminence) on the lateral side of the proximal end

surgical neck portion below the tuberosities, thus named because it is frequently the site of fractures

head large, rounded proximal end

The humerus articulates at both the proximal and distal ends. With which bones does it articulate at the proximal and distal ends?

The humerus articulates with the scapula at the proximal end and with the ulna and radius at the distal end.

Which category of bone describes the scapula?

The scapula is a flat bone, roughly triangular in shape.

Where on the scapula is the acromion located?

The acromion is a triangular projection extending anteriorly at the lateral extremity of the spine of the scapula.

What and where is the glenoid fossa?

The glenoid fossa is a shallow concavity located at the lateral angle of the scapula.

What is the spine of the scapula?

The spine of the scapula is a projecting plate of bone located at the posterior surface dividing the scapula into the supraspinous fossae.

Describe the clavicle.

The clavicle is a long, practically tubular bone, shaped somewhat like the letter S. It has a double curve and lies almost horizontally in front of the upper thorax. It articulates at the sternal end with the sternum and at the outer end with the acromion of the scapula.

What composes the proximal end of the humerus?

The head, anatomic neck, greater tuberosity, lesser tuberosity, bicipital groove, and surgical neck comprise the proximal end of the humerus.

Where and what is the bicipital groove?

The bicipital groove is a trenchlike area on the head of the humerus situated between the greater and lesser tuberosities.

What is the name of the portion of the humerus between the proximal and distal articulations?

This area is known as the shaft and is a long bone.

Where is the medial epicondyle of the humerus located?

The medial epicondyle is a bony prominence located at the distal end of the humerus on the medial side.

Describe the olecranon fossa and its location.

The olecranon fossa is a large depression located on the posterior surface of the distal end of the humerus. The olecranon process of the ulna fits into the olecranon fossa.

What is the forearm? Describe its construction.

The forearm is a part of the upper extremity and consists of two bones, the radius and ulna. They are both long bones and articulate with each other at both the proximal and distal extremities. The ulna is the longer of the two bones and is larger at the proximal end. It is located on the little finger side of the arm. The olecranon process is located on the proximal end. The radius has a rounded head located at the proximal end and is located on the thumb side of the arm. This distal end is thicker and is the site of Colles' fracture.

How many bones compose the hand?

The hand is composed of twenty-seven bones. It is divided into three parts—the wrist, the hand proper, and the five digits or fingers.

Name the bones of the wrist.

There are eight bones arranged in two rows in the wrist. Four are in the proximal row, and four are in the distal row. In the proximal row they are navicular, lunate, triangular (triquetral), and pisiform. In the distal row they are greater multangular, lesser multangular, capitate, and hamate.

Describe the bones of the palm.

Each of the five bones of the palm has a base, shaft, and head. They articulate proximally with the wrist and distally with the phalanges.

How many phalanges are there?

There are fourteen phalanges, three in each finger and two in each thumb. In the fingers they are termed proximal, middle, and distal; in the thumb they are proximal and distal.

List the bones and joints that form the elbow.

The humerus at the distal end joins from above with the proximal end of the radius and ulna from below to comprise the bones of the elbow. The areas of each that form the elbow are the coronoid fossa, capitellum, and medial and lateral epicondyle of the humerus; the head and neck at the proximal end or radioulna joint of the radius; and the coronoid process, trochlear notch, and olecranon process of the ulna.

What is the sternum?

The sternum is a long bone extending from the base of the neck to the upper abdomen and is part of the anterior thorax.

How many bones comprise the lower extremities?

There are thirty-one bones in the lower extremity, including the innominate bone of the pelvis. They are, from the top downward, innominate, femur, patella, tibia, fibula, tarsals, metatarsals, and phalanges.

The innominate bone is really three bones fused together. Name them.

The three bones fused together to form the innominate or hip bone are the ilium, ischium, and pubis. The ilium comprises the upper portion of the innominate bone. The ischium comprises the lower part of the innominate bone and has a body and superior and inferior rami. The third bone, the pubis, forms the anterior portion of the innominate bone, and it also has a body and superior and inferior rami.

Describe the acetabulum.

The acetabulum is a cup-shaped socket and the outer surface of the innominate bone. Also, it is the site of fusion of the three bones forming the innominate bone. The head of the femur fits into the acetabulum to form the hip joint.

The pelvis is comprised of two portions, the major pelvis, or false pelvis, and the true pelvis. Which areas are they?

The expanded portion above the pelvic brim is referred to as the major or false pelvis. The part of the cavity below the pelvis brim is known as the true pelvis. This area contains the bladder, rectum, and some of the reproductive organs, as well as some bowel.

How many bones comprise the sternum, and what are they?

The sternum is only about 6 to 8 inches in length and is comprised of two bones and a bony cartilage. They include the upper portion, or manubrium, which is the widest portion and articulates with the clavicles. The first pair of ribs also articulates with the manubrium. The body is the central portion and the longest of the three parts. Four pairs of ribs are located along the lateral aspect of the body. The xiphoid is the smallest and most inferior portion. It is used as a landmark at its junction with the body for the midline of the diaphragm, the upper surface of the liver, and the lower border of the heart. The seventh pair of ribs articulates with the sternum laterally at the junction of the body and xiphoid.

Which bones form the pelvis?

The pelvis is a basin-shaped ring of bone. It supports the spinal column and rests upon the lower extremities. It is made up of the two innominate bones, portions of the lumbar spine, the sacrum, and the coccyx.

What are the sacroiliac joints?

The sacroiliac joints are the junctions of the innominate bones with the sacrum. The innominate bones articulate posteriorly with the sacrum and anteriorly at the symphysis pubis.

The femur is the longest and largest bone in the body. Describe its construction and other features.

The major purpose of the femur is to transmit the weight of the body from the pelvis to the lower leg. It has a head that fits into, and articulates with, the acetabulum of the pelvis, a neck, greater and lesser trochanters, shaft, condyles, and epicondyles. It articulates at the distal end with the lower leg.

What is the patella?

The patella, or kneecap, is the largest of the sesamoid bones. It is smooth on the posterior surface and articulates with the femur.

What is the intercondylar notch?

The wide, deep groove separating the two condyles on the distal end of the femur posteriorly is the intercondylar notch.

Name the two bones in the lower leg, parallel to each other.

The two bones are named the fibula and tibia. The fibula is the smaller of the two bones and is located laterally from the tibia. It has a shaft and two extremities. The head is located on the proximal end and articulates with the tibia. The lateral malleolus is located on the distal end. The tibia is the largest of the two bones, being next in size to the femur. It has a shaft and two extremities. On the upper end (proximal) are both lateral and medial condyles and a facet for the junction of the fibula. The medial malleolus is on the distal end. The medial malleolus of the tibia and the lateral malleolus of the fibula form the ankle mortise.

How are the twenty-six bones of the foot divided?

The bones of the foot are divided into three parts—the tarsals, 7; metatarsals, 5;

and phalanges, 14. The tarsal bones articulate proximally with the tibia and fibula and distally with the metatarsal bones. The metatarsals articulate distally with the phalanges.

How are the fourteen phalanges divided?

The phalanges are divided into proximal, middle, and distal phalanx, with the exception of the great toe, which has only proximal and distal phalanges.

Name the bones of the tarsus (ankle).

The seven bones of the ankle are the talus, calcaneus, navicular, first cuneiform, second cuneiform, third cuneiform, and cuboid.

Which is the largest bone of the tarsus?

The calcaneus (os calcis) is the largest bone. It is situated beneath the astragalus and provides the shape and support of the heel.

What are the four body forms or structures?

They are the hypersthenic, sthenic, hyposthenic, and asthenic. Hypersthenic forms are strong and active, with massive builds, broad and deep thorax, wide heart, high diaphragm, and long abdomen. Sthenic forms are modified versions of the hypersthenic but not so extreme. Hyposthenic forms are rather frail and weak, having slender build, narrow and shallow thorax, long and narrow heart, low diaphragm, and short abdomen. It is not quite as extreme as asthenic forms, which have the same characteristics. The asthenic types are weak, frail, and feeble.

Into how many anatomic planes is the body divided? What are they?

The body is divided into four anatomic planes. The median plane passes in a vertical anteroposterior direction, extending through the midline of the trunk and dividing the body into two parts. The sagittal plane is parallel to the median plane. There may be many sagittal planes, each passing in a vertical anteroposterior relationship. The coronal or frontal plane is at right angles to the median plane. A transverse plane is any plane that passes in a horizontal direction at right angles to both the coronal and median planes.

How many pairs of ribs are there?

There are twelve pairs of ribs located in the thoracic cage. The first seven are connected by means of costal cartilages to the sternum. The eighth, ninth, and tenth ribs are joined to the cartilage of the seventh. The eleventh and twelfth ribs are free at the anterior extremities.

The trunk of the body is divided into two basic cavities. What are they?

The thoracic or chest cavity and the abdomen are the two basic cavities of the body. The chest cavity contains the pleural membranes, lungs, trachea, esophagus, pericardium, and heart. The abdominal cavity contains the peritoneum, gallbladder, liver, spleen, pancreas, stomach, intestines, kidneys, and ureters.

An arrangement of organs closely allied to each other and concerned with the same functions may be classified as systems. How many systems are there in the body, and what are they?

There are nine systems in the human body. They are the skeletal, muscular, nervous, vascular, endocrine, respiratory, digestive, excretory, and reproductive.

The digestive system is composed of how many parts? What are they?

The digestive system, or alimentary tract, extends about 28 feet from the mouth to the anus. It has eight parts: the mouth, pharynx, esophagus, stomach, small intestine, large intestine, rectum, and anus.

How many salivary glands are there?

There are three pairs of salivary glands—parotid, submaxillary, and sublingual. The parotid gland is situated in front of each ear; the submaxillary gland lies close to the internal surface of each half of the mandible; and the sublingual glands are located just anteriorly to the base of the tongue.

Describe the pharynx.

The pharynx is a continuation of the digestive tube behind the mouth, extending into the esophagus. It consists of three parts—the nasopharynx, oral pharynx, and laryngeal pharynx.

Describe the stomach and its component parts.

The stomach is a pear-shaped organ situated between the end of the esophagus and the beginning of the small intestine. It has an anterior and a posterior surface. The upper border is called the lesser curvature and the lower border the greater curvature. The opening at the upper end (esophagus) is the cardia. The opening into the intestine is known as the pylorus. The portion bulging upward and to the left is known as the fundus.

Name the portions of the small intestine.

The small intestine is a tube ranging from 22 to 25 feet in length, beginning at the junction of the stomach at the pylorus and ending at the ileocecal junction. It consists of the duodenum, jejunum, and ileum.

Which ducts empty into the duodenum?

The pancreatic and common bile ducts open into the duodenum.

What comprises the large intestine?

The large intestine is comprised of the cecum, ascending colon, transverse colon, descending colon, and sigmoid colon. The cecum is a blind sac located in the right iliac fossa; the ascending colon extends from the cecum to the transverse colon. It contacts the liver and is called at this juncture the hepatic flexure; the transverse colon extends from the hepatic flexure across the abdomen to the splenic flexure, so named because of the close proximity of the spleen; the descending colon turns downward in front of the left kidney to the pelvis; the sigmoid colon extends from the descending colon to the rectum.

What and where is the rectum?

The rectum is a continuation of the sigmoid colon, about 8 inches in length, passing downward (inferiorly) in the curve of the sacrum and coccyx. It terminates at the lower end, which is known as the anus.

What is the largest gland in the body?

The liver is the largest gland, located in the right hypochondrium and upper epigastric regions.

How many lobes are there in the liver?

There are two lobes, the right and left, divided by the attached falciform ligament.

What are the functions of the liver?

The functions are as follows: the secretion of bile, and metabolic functions (carbohydrate metabolism, fat metabolism, and protein metabolism).

What accessory organs are involved with digestion?

The pancreas, liver, and gallbladder are involved. The pancreas is a long organ shaped like a pistol aimed toward the hilum of the spleen. It provides a juice secreted by ducts. The liver is the largest gland and serves a variety of functions: secretion of bile, glycogenic function, and protein metabolism, to list a few. The gallbladder is a pear-shaped sac located on the undersurface of the liver in a fossa. It is a storage area for bile, and because it has involuntary muscles in the walls, is stimulated by fat to contract, forcing bile into the duodenum.

What is the appendix, and where is it located?

The appendix is a pouch located at the lower end of the cecum. It varies in length from 2 to 6 inches. The lumen of the appendix is continuous with the cecum.

Describe the kidney.

There are two kidneys, each of which is shaped like a bean. They are located in the posterior part of the abdomen, one on each side of the vertebral column and beneath the diaphragm. The right kidney is usually lower than the left. The hilum is on the medial border of each kidney, where the renal artery, vein, and pelvis enter the kidney. The ureter leaves the kidney at the hilum.

There are two ureters. What are their functions?

The ureters are two tubes leading from the kidneys to the urinary bladder. They conduct urine secreted by the kidneys to the bladder. They are approximately 10 to 12 inches in length, passing posteriorly to the abdominal wall, crossing the pelvic brim, and passing laterally to the pelvic walls and to the floor of the pelvis.

What is the urinary bladder?

The urinary bladder is a sac located in the pelvis, a reservoir for urine, which varies in size, depending upon the amount of fluid it contains.

Describe the urethra.

The urethra is the tube that conveys urine from the bladder to the exterior. In the male it is about 6 inches in length, extending from the internal urethral orifice to the end of the penis. In the female it is a narrow membranous canal, about 4 cm long, extending from the bladder to the external orifice in the vestibule. It serves

to conduct the urine from the urinary bladder to the exterior of the body.

What are the principal pathways of excretion?

These are through the skin, lungs, intestine, and kidneys. The skin excretes fluids—sweat and oil (sebum); lungs excrete carbon dioxide; intestine excretes residue of the food having escaped digestion; kidneys excrete water and urine.

What is the circulatory system?

The circulatory system is composed of the blood vascular system and the lymphatic system. It is through the blood vascular system that the blood is pumped and circulated throughout the body. The lymphatic system consists of a network of vessels and bodies that collect and transport lymph throughout the tissue spaces.

What comprises the blood vascular system?

The blood vascular system includes the heart, aorta, arteries, capillaries, and veins. The heart is the center of the circulatory system and the most vital organ of the body.

What comprises the lymphatic system?

The lacteals of the intestinal walls, lymph capillaries, lymphatic vessels, lymph nodes, and spleen comprise the lymphatic system.

Describe the heart.

The heart is divided into right and left halves, and each half is further divided by a constriction into upper and lower cavities. The upper portion is called the atrium and the lower, the ventricle. Thus, there are four chambers in the heart—right and left atria and right and left ventricles.

What are the functions of the four chambers of the heart?

The right atrium is larger than the left and has several vessels carrying blood to it. Blood is returned from the upper body by means of the superior vena cava, whereas the inferior vena cava returns blood from below or the lower portions of the body. Blood from the muscle tissue of the heart, or myocardium, is returned into the right atrium via the coronary sinus. As the blood accumulates in the right atrium, it passes into the right ventricle through the tricuspid valve. This valve consists of three segments and permits the blood to flow from the atrium to the ventricle, but normally it prevents its flow in the reverse direction during the contraction of the ventricle.

The right ventricle is the lower right cavity of the heart, which extends from the right atrium to the apex. The inner surface is marked by muscular projections that function with the heart valves. As the ventricle contracts, the blood is expelled through the pulmonary artery to the lungs. Small cuplike valves in the walls of the pulmonary artery (semilunar valves) prevent backflow of the blood. Blood from the lungs is carried to the left atrium by four pulmonary veins. From the left atrium blood is forced into the left ventricle through the left atrioventricular orifice. At this opening is located the bicuspid or mitral valve. Consisting of two segments, this valve allows the blood to flow into the left ventricle. The left ventricle is longer and more conical in shape than the right and forms the apex of the heart. The walls are very thick. The blood in the left ventricle is forced into the systemic circulation of the body through the aorta. Aortic semilunar valves (three) allow the blood to flow through the aorta from the ventricle but prevent its returning.

The heart is in continual action and must be supplied with blood to maintain its activities. What supplies the heart with blood?

Blood is supplied to the heart by the right and left coronary arteries. Veins return the blood into the coronary sinus and then into the right atrium.

What is the cardiac cycle?

The cardiac cycle consists of the phases of contraction and relaxation. The phase of contraction is called systole, whereas the phase of relaxation is called diastole.

What is pulse pressure?

The difference between the arterial systolic pressure and the diastolic pressure is called the pulse pressure.

Which nerve system supplies the heart?

The heart is under the control of the involuntary (autonomic) nervous system and an intrinsic automatic nervous system of its own. Cardiac muscular tissue possesses the power of rhythmic contractivity; that is, even if the extrinsic of external nerve supply were severed, the heart would continue to beat.

What are the capillaries?

Capillaries are the vessels that convey the blood from the arteries to the veins.

The nervous system is divided into two parts. What are they called?

The two divisions of the nervous system are the central and peripheral. Each division has elements of the autonomic nervous system. The central nervous system includes the brain and spinal cord. The peripheral nervous system includes the nerves that extend from the brain, the spinal cord, and also the more or less detached set, the autonomic nervous system.

Of what is nervous tissue composed?

Nervous tissue is composed of highly specialized tissue sensitive to stimulation, and it possesses to a high degree the property of irritability and conductivity.

What is the autonomic nervous system?

The autonomic system is that part of the nervous system that controls the activity of cardiac and smooth muscle, the sweat and digestive glands, and certain endocrine organs. The system is divided into the sympathetic and parasympathetic divisions.

The ear is divided into three parts. Name and describe them.

The three parts are the external, middle, and internal ear. The external ear, or auricle, is composed of cartilage and projects from the side of the head. It collects sound vibrations of the air, which are conducted by means of the external auditory canal to the middle ear. The middle ear is the irregular space in the temporal bone filled with air and containing the auditory ossicles—the incus, malleus, and stapes. They conduct vibrations from the tympanic membrane to the internal ear. The internal ear contains the receptors for hearing and equilibrium in relationship with the petrous portion of the temporal bone.

Of all the glands in the body, one has a more widespread effect upon the other glands and either modifies or controls their secretions. Which gland is this?

The pituitary gland is referred to as the leader. It is divided into two lobes, the anterior and posterior lobes. The anterior lobe plays the master role in its action with other glands; the posterior lobe has an effect upon the smooth muscle, causing it to contract.

Describe the brain and its component parts.

The brain, or encephalon, is the center of the nervous system. It fills the cranial cavity and is continuous with the spinal cord. The three coats of membranous tissue covering the brain are the dura mater, arachnoid, and pia mater. The two layers of matter are the gray and the white. The white matter is the innermost layer. There are three main parts of the brain and four functional parts. The three main parts are the forebrain, midbrain, and hindbrain. The forebrain contains the cerebral hemisphere; the midbrain connects the pons and cerebellum with the forebrain; and the

hindbrain is composed of the medulla oblongata, pons, and cerebellum. The functional parts are the cerebrum, cerebellum, pons, and medulla oblongata.

What are the functions of the cerebrum, cerebellum, pons, and medulla oblongata?

The cerebrum is divided into two hemispheres by fissures; these hemispheres are called ventricles. The two ventricles, called lateral ventricles, are filled with fluid. The cerebrum is also divided into lobes that are named after the bones of the cranium near which they lie. Most of the thinking and higher emotions takes place in the cerebrum.

The cerebellum is situated within the posterior part of the skull between the occipital lobes of the cerebrum. It is divided into two lateral hemispheres and a central portion, the vermis. Its principal functions are to coordinate the movements and maintain equilibrium.

The pons is a roughly shaped white mass lying in the midline of the cranial cavity at the base of the skull. It connects the midbrain with the medulla oblongata. It consists of longitudinal and transverse white fiber tracts, the former connecting the medulla oblongata with the cerebrum and the latter connecting the two halves of the cerebellum with the pons.

The medulla oblongata, or bulb of the brain, is an expanded continuation of the spinal cord, extending slightly upward and forward from the level of the foramen magnum to the pons. It conducts impulses to and from the spinal cord and brain. Many of the vital centers are contained here. Some of them and their functions are cardiac, speeding or slowing the heart rate; vasomotor, constricting or dilating the blood vessels; and respiratory, changing the rate and depth of breathing.

Describe briefly the spinal cord.

The spinal cord is approximately 18 inches long and lies in the upper two thirds of the spinal canal, extending downward to the upper border of the second lumbar vertebra. It is a part of the central nervous system and is surrounded by cerebrospinal fluid in the spinal canal.

What is cerebrospinal fluid, and how is it developed?

Cerebrospinal fluid is a clear, colorless, watery fluid that fills all the cavities in, and spaces around, the central nervous system. It is formed by the choroid plexuses in the ventricles. It is formed and drained continuously, as is tissue fluid elsewhere in the body. Cerebrospinal fluid protects the central nervous system from mechanical injury by acting as a shock absorber. It serves as a pathway for the exchange of nutrients and waste between the bloodstream and the busy cells.

Of what is cerebrospinal fluid formed?

The constituents of cerebrospinal fluid are water, glucose, potassium, sodium chloride, traces of protein, and a few white blood cells. It has a specific gravity of 1.004 to 1.008. The quantity of cerebrospinal fluid varies with individuals, but the average amount in adults is between 100 and 200 ml.

Trace the flow or pathway of the cerebrospinal fluid from the lateral ventricles.

The cerebrospinal fluid leaves the elongated lateral ventricles via a narrow, oval opening, the foramen of Monro, and proceeds into the third ventricle, which is a slitlike cavity located between the right and left thalami; from the third ventricle it passes through the aqueduct of Sylvius into the fourth ventricle, which is a diamond-shaped cavity located between the medulla oblongata and the pons anteriorly and the cerebellum posteriorly. From the fourth ventricle the cerebrospinal fluid flows via three openings into the cranial subarachnoid space. Two openings are the foramina of Magendie. From the cranial subarachnoid space the fluid flows around the spinal cord and brain and is drained by filtration.

How many nerves are there to the cranium, and what are they called?

There are twelve pairs of cranial nerves originating from the undersurface of the brain. Most of them are classified as mixed nerves, having both motor and sensory fibers. Three pairs contain only sensory components (olfactory, optic, and acoustic). They are the olfactory, optic, oculomotor, trochlear, trigeminal, abducens, facial, acoustic, glossopharyngeal, vagus, accessory, and hypoglossal nerves.

The olfactory nerves conduct impulses related to the sense of smell. Optic nerves are the nerves of vision. Oculomotor nerves control eye movement. Trochlear nerves supply motor and sensory fibers to the superior oblique muscles of the eye on its own side. The trigeminal nerves are referred to as the great sensory nerves of the head and face, with the sensory portion of each consisting of three divisions—ophthalmic, maxillary, and mandibular. The abducen nerves supply both motor and sensory fibers to the lateral rectus muscle of the eye on its own side. The facial nerves supply efferent fibers to all muscles concerned with facial expression. Acoustic nerves are concerned with hearing and equilibrium. Glossopharyngeal central nerves are concerned with the tongue and the pharynx. Vagus nerves, after arising from the medulla, live up to their name, which means "wanderer." Each vagus nerve contains both somatic and visceral fibers; they supply the organs in the neck, thorax, and abdomen. Accessory nerves supply somatic and sensory fibers to the sternocleidomastoid and part of the trapezius muscles. The hypoglossal nerves supply motor and sensory fibers to the muscles of the tongue. They are important in speech, mastication, and deglutition.

Which arteries supply the head with blood?

The arteries arising from the arch of the aorta and supplying blood to the head, neck, and upper extremities are the innominate, left common carotid, and left subclavian arteries. The innominate is the largest of the arteries, but it divides into the right common carotid and the right subclavian arteries. The right and left common carotid arteries bifurcate at the level of the upper border of the thyroid cartilage into an external and an internal carotid artery. The external carotid artery has branches called superficial temporal and internal maxillary; the internal carotid artery also has branches, the ophthalmic, posterior communicating, and anterior and middle cerebral.

What is the circle of Willis, and how is it formed?

The circle of Willis is an arterial anastomosis at the base of the brain. The anterior part is formed by the anterior cerebral arteries, branches of the internal carotid, which are connected by the anterior communicating artery. Posteriorly it is formed by the two posterior cerebral arteries, branches of the basilar, which are connected on either side with the internal carotid by the posterior communicating artery.

What are ductless glands? Name them and their functions.

Ductless glands are those organs whose function is to produce special secretions containing hormones, which are discharged into the blood or lymph. They are further classified as the endocrine system and as glands of internal secretion. They are individual glands located in widely separated regions of the body and form a system only from a functional standpoint. The hormones secreted by these glands excite associated organs to activity. The glands are the spleen, pineal, pituitary, thyroid, parathyroids, thymus, and suprarenals. The functions of the spleen are to produce blood and fight disease. The pineal is located above and behind the pituitary and is necessary for the proper development of the eyeballs. The pituitary hangs from the undersurface of the brain and is protected by the sella turcica. It is divided into two lobes, the posterior and anterior. The anterior lobe secretes hormones affecting thyroid metabolism, carbohydrate metabolism, sex, and growth. The posterior lobe secretes hormones for controlling the blood pressure and constricting arteries. The thyroid also has two lobes, one on each side of the larynx. It secretes thyroxin and has a definite influence on body growth and nervous stability. The parathyroids are located two on each side of the thyroid, and their secretions regulate calcium metabolism, which is important in bones, blood, and other tissues. The thymus is located behind the sternum, and its secretions affect body growth and the development of reproductive organs. The suprarenals are two glands, one on the upper pole of each kidney. Each gland has two portions, the medulla and cortex. The medulla, or inner portion, secretes adrenaline and regulates temperature as well as blood pressure. The cortex secretions regulate water and salt metabolism.

Define briefly the male reproductive system.

The male reproductive system consists of ten main parts: the testes, epididymis, ductus deferens, seminal vesicle, ejaculatory duct, bulbourethral gland, prostate, scrotum, penis, and urethra.

The two testes, suspended from the inguinal region, produce sperm cells and male hormones. The epididymis are also two in number and unite to form a single tube that joins the ductus deferens. There are two ductus deferens extending up the posterior surface of the testicle through the inguinal canal to the inferior end of the seminal vesicle; the ejaculatory duct extends from the seminal vesicle and ductus deferens junction to the prostatic portion of the urethra. The seminal vesicles are two in number and are situated between the rectum and urinary bladder; they are reservoirs for semen. The bulbourethral, or Cowper's, glands are two small bodies the size of the pea, located one on each side of the membranous urethra, and they secrete a fluid that forms part of the seminal fluid; the prostate surrounds the upper portion of the urethra and secretes a fluid to keep sperm mobile. The scrotum is a muscular, membranous sac that surrounds and supports the testicles. The penis consists of three somewhat cylindrical bodies composed largely of erectile tissue. The portion forming the distal end is called the glans penis; the thin layer of skin extending down over the glans penis is called the prepuce. The urethra is a tube extending from the urinary bladder to the meatus of the penis; it is a passageway for semen as well as urine.

Define the female reproductive system.

The female genital organs are divided into five main parts: ovaries, uterus, fallopian tubes, vagina, and clitoris.

The ovaries are two in number, corresponding to the testes in the male, and form the egg or ovum. The uterus is located between the urinary bladder and rectum, behind the symphysis pubis in the midline. The fundus portion is free, and the cervix portion is located at the vaginal end. The body portion is between the fundus and cervix; the fallopian tubes, uterine tubes or oviducts, extend down from the ovaries and carry the ovum downward so that conception may take place. The vagina is a passageway about 3 inches long leading to the lower end of the uterus from the vulva or external portion. The clitoris is the morphologic equivalent of the penis of the male. It is a small elongated, erectile body situated at the anterior angle of the vulva.

What are the parts comprising the respiratory system?

The respiratory system consists of the lungs and air passages leading into them. They may be divided into those concerned with external aspiration and with internal respiration. External respiration involves the exchange of gases between the circulating blood and the air. The internal respiration involves the exchange of gases between the circulating blood and the various tissue cells as they use oxygen and produce waste carbon dioxide. The organs concerned with external respiration are the nose, pharynx, larynx, trachea, bronchi, and lungs. The lungs are the essential organs of respiration, and it is here that the exchange of gases between the blood and air takes place. They are two in number and occupy most of the area in the thoracic cavity. The portion of the lung receiving the bronchus, blood vessels, and nerves is called the hilum. The lungs are composed of bronchial tubes, alveoli, blood vessels, lymphatics, nerves, and connective tissue. A delicate serous membrane, the pleura, envelops each lung.

REFERENCES

Jacobi, C.: Textbook of anatomy and physiology in radiologic technology, St. Louis, 1968, The C. V. Mosby Co.

Lockhart, R. D., Hamilton, G. F., and Fyfe, F. W.: Anatomy of the human body, Philadelphia, 1969, J. B. Lippincott Co.

Mallett, M.: A handbook of anatomy and physiology for the student x-ray technician, Ann Arbor, Mich., 1962, Edwards Brothers, Inc.

Ville, C.: Biology, Philadelphia, 1967, W. B. Saunders Co.

7 NURSING PROCEDURES

Who are the members of the health team?

The physician, nurse, and technicians (laboratory, x-ray) are members of the immediate health team. Every person involved in the treatment and care of illness is considered a member of the team.

When moving a patient from a stretcher to an x-ray table, what is the most important principle to remember?

The important principle is to lock the wheels of the stretcher so that it will not move while the patient is being transferred to the table.

Is there a correct way to move the patient?

Yes. After explaining clearly what is desired, always allow the patient to assist if he is able to do so. If the patient is unable to assist, then the technologist should roll, push, or slide the patient rather than lift him.

What is the most common emergency in the x-ray department?

The most common emergency is syncope. This is a partial or complete temporary suspension of respiration and circulation caused by cerebral ischemia.

What is insulin shock?

Insulin shock is the condition of the body when carbohydrates are needed.

If a patient is brought into the x-ray department with a question of a fractured cervical vertebra, should the patient be moved to the table?

Unless the patient is on a stretcher that would allow placing over the table and lowering to the table he should not be moved. Otherwise, films should be taken on the stretcher without any unnecessary movement.

If a patient states that he is feeling faint, what procedure should be followed?

A patient feeling faint should be allowed to lie down, and any tight-fitting garments should be loosened.

In preparing a patient's skin for a procedure necessitating either injection or cutdown, what procedures should be followed?

To ensure that the area is free from all bacteria-producing disease, cleanse it by starting at the center of the area and, with a circular motion, working outward.

What is a main principle of sterile technique?

Never turn your back on a sterile field after it has been cleansed or sterilized.

If a patient begins to have convulsions while in the department, what should be done?

Gentle restraint should be applied, and every precaution should be taken to prevent the patient from swallowing his tongue.

When performing artificial respiration during closed external massage, what should be the rate of thrusts?

The rate should be about sixty thrusts per minute.

A patient in shock will usually show changes in blood pressure. How will it react?

The blood pressure of a patient in shock will decrease.

Before commencing any type of artificial respiration, what should be done?

First clean out the patient's mouth with your fingers.

What could be a symptom of internal bleeding?

Restlessness on the part of the patient could indicate internal bleeding.

If a patient is suspected of bleeding from the venous system, what is the best way to combat it?

The most effective way would be to apply direct pressure to the site of bleeding.

What important information should the technologist know about his x-ray department?

He should know the emergency procedure to be followed in the event that one arises and where the emergency equipment and drugs are kept.

A patient is brought into the x-ray department and suspected of having a skull fracture. What visible signs are there, if any?

If unequal pupils are found to exist upon investigation of the patient, this is a good indication of a skull fracture.

What are the differences between disinfection and sterilization?

Disinfection is the killing of disease-producing or pathogenic bacteria—not all bacteria. Sterilization means the killing of all bacteria, disease-producing or otherwise, and is usually accomplished by boiling or autoclaving for a specified time.

Should anesthetized or unconscious patients be left in any position?

Patients who are either anesthetized or unconscious should be kept in a position lying on their side.

A patient in a diabetic coma would have what symptoms?

A patient in a diabetic coma would have hot, dry, flushed skin, and his breath would have a sweetish odor.

What are the differences between shock and hemorrhage?

Shock is a condition in which all the body activities are greatly depressed, with a consequent "pooling" of blood in the abdomen, which is away from the vital centers of heart and brain. Hemorrhage is the escape of blood from one or more blood vessels of the body, arteries, veins, or capillaries. A patient in shock from hemorrhage is weak, faint, and restless.

When preparing a patient for an examination involving injections of contrast media, should he be informed?

When a patient must undergo an examination involving a contrast medium, the chances of ill effects are always possible, and the patient should be informed that he may feel flushed, become slightly nauseous, or perhaps have a choking sensation. This will alert him to the possible effects, and if nothing occurs, he is relieved.

Certain precautions must be followed when injections are to be given. What are they?

One should be sure he has the right patient, right drug, right amount, and right time. An injection will allow the material to enter the bloodstream much faster than one taken orally and has more serious complications.

Should surgical dressings be removed for x-ray examinations?

Surgical dressings are not removed usually since the gauze, bandage, and pads are not opaque and will not require removal. When barium enemas through colostomies are being done, the bandages must be removed since surgery has been performed on the rectum and small bowel.

What are some precautions to be followed by technologists to assist in preventing the spread of disease?

Careful washing of the hands between care of patients, turning one's head to cough or sneeze into a handkerchief, providing clean sheets and pillowcases for every patient, wearing clean uniforms, and maintaining general good hygiene are precautions in preventing the spread of disease.

8 RADIOGRAPHIC POSITIONING

What two main groups divide the bony framework of the body?

The body is divided into the appendicular skeleton, consisting of the upper and lower extremities, the shoulders, and the pelvis and the axial skeleton, consisting of the skull, the vertebral column, the sternum, and the ribs.

Describe the anatomic position and the planes of the body.

The anatomic position is described as the body erect, with the arms by the sides and with the palms turned out.

The median, or midsagittal, plane is a line that passes vertically through the body from front to back, dividing the body into equal left and right halves.

The coronal, or frontal, plane is a line that passes vertically through the midaxillary portion of the body from side to side and divides the body into anterior and posterior portions.

The transverse, or horizontal, plane is a line that passes crosswise through the body at right angles to the longitudinal axis and divides the body into superior and inferior segments.

Define the following terms in relation to location and position: anterior, posterior, superior, inferior, medial, lateral, proximal, and distal.

anterior refers to the forward part of the body. The word "ventral" also may be used to denote the same meaning.

posterior refers to the back part, or rear, of the body. The word "dorsal" may be used instead.

superior refers to parts or direction toward the head of the body. Toward the head may also be designated by the use of cephalic.

inferior refers to those parts away from the head and toward the feet. Caudal direction refers to parts toward the feet.

medial refers to parts and positions toward the midline of the body.

lateral refers to those parts away from the midline of the body either in the right or left direction.

proximal refers to the upper part of an extremity or that which is closest to the source.

distal refers to the part that is farthest away from the anatomic source or the lower end of an extremity.

Name and define terms that describe body positions.

supine lying on the back
prone lying face down or on the stomach
recumbent lying down
decubitus usually associated with lying on the side
supinate palm turned up
pronate palm turned down
evert to turn part outward
invert to turn part inward
extension to straighten the joint

abduct to move the part away from the midline of the body

adduct to move the part toward the midline of the body.

left lateral decubitus lying on the left side.

In the posteroanterior view of the hand are all the bones viewed in the posteroanterior projection?

No. All the bones are shown in the posteroanterior projection except the thumb, which this view shows in an oblique view.

What position should be taken to correct the foreshortening of the navicular?

The view to correct the navicular foreshortening is the posteroanterior view of the wrist with ulnar flexion. The wrist is positioned as it would be for a posteroanterior view. The wrist is held in position and the elbow moved away from the body slightly. The hand is turned outward until the wrist is in extreme ulnar flexion.

What projections or positions of the wrist best demonstrate the pisiform, cuneiform, and hamate?

These wrist bones are best demonstrated by radiographing the part in the anteroposterior oblique position. The wrist is placed either in the lateral or the supinated position on the film holder. The wrist is then rotated so that it forms a 45-degree angle to the plane of the film.

Describe the position of the wrist to demonstrate the navicular using the Stecher position.

The patient's wrist is placed in the posteroanterior position on a film holder that has been angled 20 degrees toward the patient. The wrist joint is centered to the film. The central ray is directed perpendicular to the plane of the table and through the navicular bone.

Stecher says that the same view can be obtained by placing the wrist prone on the table and centering it to the film. The central ray is directed 20 degrees toward the elbow entering at the site of the navicular.

How would you position the patient to radiograph the carpal canal?

The patient is seated at the end of the table with the forearm and wrist placed in pronation. The wrist is hyperextended, and the hand is placed so that the long axis is vertical to the table. The wrist is placed upon the film and the radial styloid centered to the midpoint. The hand is rotated slightly toward the radius. If necessary, the patient is asked to hold the extended fingers in the vertical position. The central ray is directed toward the palm at a 25-degree angle and enters the wrist one inch distal to the base of the fourth metatarsal.

When using the anteroposterior view of the forearm, the technologist should remember what important factor?

The technologist must remember to have the hand supinated. Pronation of the hand in this view crosses the radius over the ulna at its upper one third. In addition, the humerus is rotated medially.

What conditions should exist to obtain a lateral view of the elbow?

The following conditions should exist to obtain a lateral view of the elbow:
1. The elbow should be flexed 90 degrees.
2. The upper arm should be in the same plane as the lower arm.
3. The hand must be adjusted to the lateral position.
4. The humeral epicondyles must be perpendicular to the plane of the film.

How would you radiograph the foot to show the tarsus and the subtalar joint?

Of the many views to be taken to show this anatomy, the lateromedial oblique projection described by Feist and Mankin is best.

The patient is placed in the seated position on the table. The leg is flexed and rotated medially so that the long axis of the leg forms a 45-degree angle to the plane of the film. The leg is supported with angle blocks. The medial aspect of the foot is placed on the film, and a 45-degree angle support is placed underneath the elevated side. The central ray is directed perpendicular to the film, passing through the lateral aspect of the foot at a point just distal to the lateral malleolus.

What advantages are there to radiographing the lateral ankle with the medial side in contact with the film?

With the patient in this position the ankle joint is closer to the film and provides considerable improvement in the projected image. The ankle is also positioned more exactly and more consistently when the joint is resting on the flat surface of the medial side.

What difference is there in the direction of the central ray when radiographing the knee to show the joint space and the distal end of the femur?

When radiographing the joint space, the central ray is directed 7 degrees toward the head. When radiographing the distal end of the femur or the proximal end of the tibia and fibula the central ray is directed perpendicular to the joint space.

In the lateral projection of the knee why is the central ray directed 5 degrees toward the head?

When the central ray is angled 5 degrees toward the head, the slight angulation will prevent the joint space from being obscured by the medial femoral condyle in its magnified projection.

Describe the views that show the intercondyloid fossa.

The following projections may be taken to show the intercondyloid fossa.

The Camp-Coventry position places the patient in the prone position on the table, with no rotation of the body. The affected leg is raised, and the foot is placed on supports so that the lower leg forms a 40-degree angle with the upper leg. The proximal half of the cassette is centered to the knee joint. The central ray is directed perpendicular to the long axis of the leg (40 degrees) and enters the posterior portion of the knee at the popliteal depression.

In the Béclère position the patient is placed supine on the table with no rotation of the body. The knee is flexed so that the femur forms a 60-degree angle with the lower leg. The knee is supported on sandbags. The cassette (curved or flexible film holder) is placed under the knee and centered to the central ray. The central ray is directed through the knee joint perpendicular to the long axis of the lower leg.

The Holmblad position places the patient on the table in the kneeling position with the feet extending over the edge of the table. The patient leans forward on his hands so that the femur forms a 70-degree angle to the plane of the film. The film is centered to the lower edge of the patella. The central ray is directed perpendicular to the center of the film.

What views are taken of any anatomic part?

The technologist should take two views of the anatomic part, each view at right angles to each other to secure proper perspective and relation of the parts to the surrounding tissues.

What positions would be used to view the sternum?

For the posteroanterior oblique view of the sternum the patient is placed prone on the table, with the median plane centered to the midline of the table. The body is rotated into the right posterior oblique position and adjusted so that the sternum is free from superimposition of the dorsal spine. The film is centered to the midportion of the sternum. The central ray is directed perpendicular to the film and through the sternum.

For the lateral view the patient is placed in the lateral position with the arms behind the back, and the sternum is placed in the midline of the table. The film is centered to the midportion of the sternum (halfway between the sternal notch and the inferior tip of the xiphoid process). The central ray is directed perpendicular to the film and centered to the middle of the film.

What position would be used to radiograph the sternoclavicular articulations?

For a radiograph of the sternoclavicular articulation in the posteroanterior projection the patient is placed prone on the table, with the median plane centered to the midline of the table. The arms are placed alongside the patient's body, and the shoulders are adjusted to lie in the same plane. To show both articulations the patient's head is resting on the chin; to show only one articulation the patient is asked to rotate his head toward the affected side and to rest his head on his cheek. The film is centered to the spinous process of the third vertebra. The central ray is directed perpendicular to the film.

In the posteroanterior oblique position the patient is placed prone on the table, and then the body is adjusted in the oblique position to project the vertebral shadows behind the joint. The sternal joint is placed in the midline of the table and the film centered to it. The central ray is directed perpendicular to the film through the joint.

What instructions relative to breathing would you give the patient when radiographing the ribs?

If the radiographic examination was for the ribs below the diaphragm, the patient would be instructed to hold his breath after exhalation. For ribs above the diaphragm the breathing is stopped at full inhalation.

What views may be considered essential in radiography for suspected fracture of the ribs?

In a suspected fracture of the ribs a posteroanterior or anteroposterior view of the questionable area would be taken. The particular projection would depend upon the site of injury. In addition, both oblique views of the area could be taken. Some routines suggest that a posteroanterior chest view done in the upright position also be included.

Describe the Cleaves position for the femoral necks.

The Cleaves position, popularly known as the frog position, is performed with the patient placed supine on the table and with the median plane centered to the midline of the table. The patient is asked to flex his hips and knees and to draw his feet up as far as possible. The thighs are then abducted and the patient's feet turned inward with the soles of the feet braced against one another. The thighs are abducted from 35 to 40 degrees from the vertical position and thus place the femoral necks parallel with the plane of the film.

Describe the position for the lateral view of the femoral neck.

The patient is placed supine on the table. To localize the long axis of the femoral neck, a line is drawn from the anterosuperior iliac spine to the upper border of the symphysis pubis, and the center is marked. A second line is drawn from the center of this first line to a point 1 inch distal to the lateral projection of the greater trochanter. This line will parallel the long axis of the femoral neck. The uninjured part is raised out of the way and supported. The cassette is placed in the vertical position with the upper border in contact with, or slightly above, the iliac crest. The lower border is drawn away from the body and placed so that it parallels the femoral neck. The central ray is directed perpendicular to the femoral neck and enters the thigh about 2 inches below the intersection of the localizing lines.

The "chewing view" is associated with what anatomic part? How is it accomplished?

The chewing view is a method employed to visualize the entire cervical spine on one radiograph. The patient is placed supine on the table, with the median plane centered to the midline of the table and perpendicular to it. The head is adjusted so that the edges of the upper central incisor teeth are vertical with the mastoid tips. The head is immobilized with a head clamp. The film is centered to the fourth cervical vertebra. The central ray is directed to the center of the film. During the exposure the patient is asked to open and close his mouth rapidly. The motion of the mandible will obliterate the shadow of the structure, and all the cervical vertebrae will be seen.

All factors, considering position and direction of central ray, being as they are, what important fact must be considered in radiography of the oblique cervical spine?

In radiography of the oblique cervical spine it is important to realize what foramina are being visualized on the finished film. Radiography of the cervical spine in the posteroanterior oblique projection demonstrates the foramina closest to the film. The foramina farthest away from the film are demonstrated by the anteroposterior oblique projection.

In radiography of the entire dorsal spine why is it desirable to place the patient's head at the anode end of the tube?

With the patient in this position the greatest concentration of radiation caused by the "heel effect" is directed toward the thickest region of the dorsal vertebrae. This results in a more uniform density of the dorsal spine.

What is the "twining" position, which is used to demonstrate the cervicothoracic spines?

The patient is placed in a lateral position before an upright Bucky. The patient may stand or be seated. The midaxillary line is centered to the midline of the Bucky.

Raise the patient's arm nearest the film and rest the forearm on top of his head. Rotate his shoulder slightly forward or backward. The shoulder remote from the film is rotated in the opposite direction and depressed by having the patient hold a sandbag. Remember that the purpose of this double rotation is to prevent superimposition of the shoulders upon the vertebrae. The patient's body should not be rotated.

The film is centered to the second dorsal vertebra, and the central ray is directed at right angles to the film and to its midpoint. If the patient's shoulder is not well-depressed, the central ray is directed 5 degrees toward his feet and to the midpoint of the film.

Describe the "swimming view" for the cervicothoracic region.

The patient is placed laterally recumbent on the table with the midaxillary line centered to the midline of the table. The cervical and dorsal vertebrae are adjusted to be parallel with the plane of the table. The knees are flexed. The arm closest to the table is raised directly over the head. The patient holds a sandbag attached to a string and allowed to hang over the end of the table. The upper arm is depressed by having the patient grasp a string attached to the foot and the legs, extended slightly from the flexed position. If this is not possible, a sandbag attached to a string and hung over the table end can be utilized.

The film is centered to the second dorsal vertebra. The central ray is angled 5 degrees to the feet and is directed to the midpoint of the film.

Are there advantages to radiographing the lumbar spine in the posteroanterior projection?

If we consider the comfort of the patient as an advantage, it is beneficial. The patient with a painful back and the emaciated patient are grateful for this consideration.

However, since the posteroanterior position places the spine in a concave position, the disk spaces now nearly parallel the divergence of the x-ray beam from the tube.

Why is it important to flex the knees when radiographing the lumbar spine in the anteroposterior projection?

With the patient lying in the supine position on the table, his back remains fully arched. The position accentuates the lordotic curve of the spine, which increases the angle of the vertebral bodies and the x-ray beam. This results in distortion of the bodies and poor visualization of the disk spaces. The normal curvature of the back can be reduced by having the patient flex his knees.

Explain the so-called butterfly position for examination of the sacroiliac joints.

The patient is placed supine on the table with the median plane centered to the midline of the table. The lower extremities are extended. The central ray is directed 35 degrees to the head through the lumbosacral joint and centered to the midpoint of the film.

In radiographing the sacrum and coccyx, in what direction is the central ray angled?

For radiographing the sacrum, if the patient is radiographed in the anteroposterior projection the central ray is angled 15 degrees toward the head. If the patient is done in the prone position, the central ray is angled 15 degrees toward the feet.

When radiographing the coccyx in the anteroposterior position, the central ray is directed 10 degrees toward the feet. The prone position demands a 10-degree angulation to the head.

What effect, if any, do inspiration and expiration have in radiography of the sternum, lumbar and thoracic spine, and ribs?

In all radiographic views of the lateral thoracic spine, oblique sternum, and ribs above the diaphragm films made on inspiration will require less x-ray exposure than those made on expiration because part opacity will be less. Films of the anteroposterior lumbar spine and the ribs below the diaphragm will require more exposure if made on inspiration than on expiration.

Describe the position for radiography of the spine of the ischium.

The patient is placed supine on the table. The body is then rotated from the supine position to the side opposite the part being examined until the body is in a semilateral (45-degree) position. The median plane of the body is placed on the midline of the table. The x-ray tube is angled 15 degrees toward the feet, with the central ray directed to a point on the median plane, halfway between the superior margin of the pubis symphysis and the level of the anterosuperior iliac spine. This film is centered to the central ray.

In radiography of the lateral cervical spine, which is done in the erect position, why is the focal film distance usually 72 inches?

Because of the excessive object-film distance of the cervical spine, there will be magnification and loss of radiographic detail of the vertebral shadows. Increasing the distance to 72 inches minimizes the magnification and decreases the penumbra effect.

What is the dorsoventral view of the hand?

The dorsoventral view of the hand is the posteroanterior view. It is obtained by placing the hand palm down on the film and directing the central ray through the back of the hand.

Which position best shows the spaces between the articular surface of the patella and the femur?

The lateral projection of the knee is best.

What projections would you perform to secure a "skyline" view of the patella?

The "skyline" or axial view for the patella may be performed in either the supine or the prone position. In the supine view the knee is flexed so that the patella is at right angles to the film. The film is placed on the lower end of the femur and centered to the patella. The film is either strapped in position or held in position by the patient. The central ray is directed to the midportion of the film at right angles to the joint space between the patella and femoral condyles.

With the patient in the prone position he is asked to flex his knee as much as possible. If the knee is painful to the patient, it should be flexed slowly until the desired position is reached. The patella should be at right angles to the film. A long piece of string, tape, or bandage is looped around the patient's ankle and then given to the patient to hold the leg into position. The film is centered to the patella, and the central ray is directed to the midportion of the film at right angles to the joint space between the patella and femoral condyles.

What part of the anatomy should be radiographed for a suspected fracture of the lateral malleolus?

The ankle should be radiographed in the anteroposterior, lateral, and oblique or mortise views to demonstrate a fracture of the lateral malleolus.

What landmarks should be used and to what points should they be centered in the following examinations?

Elbow. Landmark is the epicondyles; centering is to a point midway between the epicondyles.

Knee. Landmarks are the patella and the condyles of the femur; centering is to the lower border of the patella and a point midway between the condyles.

Pelvis. Landmarks are the anterosuperior spines and the pubic symphysis; centering is to a point midway between these two landmarks.

Shoulder. Landmark is the coracoid process; centering is to the coracoid process.

Atlas and axis (open mouth). Landmark is the superimposition of the open-mouth central incisor teeth over the lower edge of mastoid tips; the centering point is through the midpoint of the open mouth.

Lumbar spine. Landmark is the iliac crest; the centering point is through the third lumbar vertebra.

Define the following radiographic base lines: glabellomeatal line, orbitomeatal line, infraorbitomeatal line, and acanthiomeatal line.

glabellomeatal line a line drawn from the external auditory meatus to the glabella

orbitomeatal (radiographic) base line a line drawn from the outer canthus of the eye to the external auditory meatus

infraorbitomeatal (Reid's) base line a line drawn from the inferior margin of the orbit to the external auditory meatus

acanthiomeatal line a line drawn from the acanthian to the external auditory meatus

Describe the classifications of the skull.

There are three major classifications of the skull:

Mesocephalic skull, which more or less corresponds to the average skull. The internal structures of the skull lie in a 47-degree plane with relation to the median plane.

Dolichocephalic skull, which is long from front to back, narrow from side to side, and deep from vertex to base.

The internal structures form a 40-degree angle with the median plane.

Brachiocephalic skull, which is formed short from front to back, wide from side to side, and shallow from vertex to base. The internal structures form a 54-degree angle with the median plane.

In the posteroanterior view of the skull what modifications of the central ray may be used and why?

In radiographing the skull in the posteroanterior projection the central ray may be directed 15 degrees toward the feet for a general survey film of the cranium. The degree of angulation will vary as do the different techniques in hospitals; the central ray is directed perpendicular to the film and passes through the nasion for a view of the frontal bone, and the central ray is directed from 20 to 25 degrees toward the feet when the superior orbital fissures need to be demonstrated.

Describe the Towne's view of the skull.

The patient is placed in the supine position or seated erect. The median plane is centered to the midline of the table. The patient's head is positioned so that the orbitomeatal line is at right angles to the film. The uppermost part of the cassette is placed at the vertex of the skull. The central ray is directed at a 35-degree, caudad angle and passes through the foramen magnum. This view shows the occipital bone.

What views of the skull will show the dorsum sellae and posterior clinoid processes?

The dorsum sellae and posterior clinoid processes may be demonstrated by placing the patient supine on the table and adjusting the head so that the infraorbitomeatal line is perpendicular to the table. The central ray is directed 37 degrees toward the feet through the foramen magnum.

In the Haas position the patient is placed prone on the table with the orbitomeatal line perpendicular to the film. The central ray is directed 25 degrees toward the head. It enters the skull 2 inches below the inion and emerges 2 inches above the nasion. This view shows the dorsum sellae and posterior clinoid processes through the foramen magnum.

To project the dorsum sellae and posterior clinoid processes through the frontal bone, the patient is placed prone on the table with the orbitomeatal line perpendicular to the midline of the table. The central ray is directed 10 degrees to the head through the glabella.

What is the Law position in radiography of the mastoids?

The Law position in radiography of the mastoids is done in the lateral projection. The patient's head is placed in a true lateral position with the median plane parallel to the plane of the film, and the interpupillary line is perpendicular to the film. Both ears are taped forward. The central ray is directed 15 degrees toward the feet and 15 degrees toward the anterior face. It enters the skull 2 inches above and 2 inches posterior to the external auditory meatus closest to the tube.

The modified Law view may be used rather than the double angulation of the tube. In this projection the patient's head is placed so that it assumes an angle of 15 degrees toward the film. The central ray is directed 15 degrees toward the feet and enters the skull 2 inches above and 2 inches posterior to the external auditory meatus closest to the tube.

Describe the examination of the petrous portion of the temporal bone using the Stenvers position.

With the patient placed in the prone position, the median plane is centered to the midline of the table. The patient's head is adjusted so that the median plane forms a 45-degree angle with the plane of the film and the head is resting on the forehead, nose, and zygoma. The central ray is directed 12 degrees toward the head and is directed through the auditory meatus closest to the film.

What is the Caldwell position for the paranasal sinuses?

The Caldwell position for the paranasal sinuses is used for the demonstration of the frontal and anterior ethmoid sinuses. The patient is placed prone or seated erect with the nasion in the center of the film. The glabellomeatal line is perpendicular to the film, and the patient's head is resting on the forehead and nose. The central ray is directed 23 degrees toward the feet and emerges through the glabella.

In the modified Caldwell projection the orbitomeatal line is placed perpendicular to the plane of the film. The nasion is centered to the middle of the film with the patient's head resting on the forehead and nose. The central ray is directed 15 degrees toward the feet and emerges through the glabella.

What position of the skull will best demonstrate the maxillary sinuses?

The Waters position of the skull will best demonstrate the maxillary sinuses. The patient may be placed prone or seated erect, with the median plane centered to the midportion of the cassette or table. The head is resting on the nose and chin. Adjust the patient's head by raising the nose off the film so that the orbitomeatal line forms a 37-degree angle with the plane of the film. The central ray is directed perpendicular to the film, enters the skull at the vertex, and emerges at the anterior nasal spine.

Why is the Waters projection done with a 37-degree angle?

To most adequately show the maxillary sinuses, the pars petrosae should be placed below the antral floor. When the head is

angled less than 37 degrees, the shadows of the petrosae will lie in the lower areas of the antra. When the head is overextended, the antra are foreshortened and the antral floors are obscured. In the early days of radiography the nose was placed so that it assumed a position of 0.5 to 1.5 cm. from the film. Technologists used their fingers to judge the correct angulation. However, this process was superseded in 1930 by H. O. Mahoney, who demonstrated that the majority of subjects were best radiographed by placing the orbitomeatal line at a 37-degree angle to the film.

What views are considered to be adequate for an examination of the skull?

The positions considered to be adequate for an examination of the skull would include the posteroanterior, anteroposterior, lateral, occipital, and inferosuperior or superoinferior (basal) view. All these may be done in stereo pairs if so desired. In cases of extreme inability of the patient to cooperate, the basal views may be omitted until a later date.

If only one view of the facial bones could be performed to demonstrate questionable fracture, which one would be most applicable?

The general survey film most desired to demonstrate questionable fractures of the facial bones would be the Waters position with some modification. The patient is placed in the same position as for the sinus projection except that the orbitomeatal line forms a 40-degree angle with the plane of the film. The central ray is directed to the center of the film through the acanthion.

In determining the presence or absence of a fracture of the zygomatic arch, what two views may be used?

One view may be the submentovertical projection. The patient is placed supine on the table or seated erect. The median plane is perpendicular to the tabletop. The head is extended until the orbitomeatal line is parallel to the plane of the table. In the supine position it may be necessary to place some pads under the patient's back to allow extension of the head. The head is resting on the vertex. Direct the central ray at right angles to the orbitomeatal line, and center it to the midpoint of the zygomatic arches. The film is centered to the central ray. The technique will have to be adjusted from the basal view technique. This view shows both arches projected free from the other structures.

The second projection might be the semiaxial or the modified Towne's view. The patient is placed in the same position as for a Towne's view of the skull. The film is centered to the mandibular angles. The central ray is directed toward the feet at a 30-degree angle and enters the skull at the glabella.

How is the patient positioned for radiographing the temporomandibular joints?

To show the temporomandibular articulations the patient's head is placed in the lateral position. This may be done with the patient in the semiprone position on the table or seated at an upright Bucky. The head is placed in the true lateral position with the median plane parallel to the plane of the film and the interpupillary line perpendicular to it. The temporomandibular articulation, usually found ½ inch anterior and 1 inch superior to the external auditory meatus, is placed in the center of the film. The central ray is directed from 30 to 35 degrees toward the feet and enters the skull through the upper parietal region and emerges through the articulation closest to the film. Two films are taken, the first with the patient's mouth closed and the next with the patient's mouth open wide. Both temporomandibular joints are taken for comparison. It is wise to have available a cork or some

other suitable material to place in the patient's mouth during the open-mouth view. This ensures both views with the same degree of opening. Whenever possible, this projection should be done in the Bucky or should utilize a tunnel arrangement to ensure the patient remaining in the same position during the examination.

Discuss the examination of the salivary ducts by means of sialography.

Sialography is the radiographic examination of the salivary glands after the injection of opaque medium. This examination demonstrates the relationship of the salivary glands to the adjacent structures.

What landmarks are used and to what points are they centered in the following examinations?

Sella turcica (lateral). Landmark is the external auditory meatus; the centering point is 1 inch above and 1 inch anterior to the external auditory meatus.

Optic foramen. Landmarks are the forehead, nose, and zygoma in the three-point landing; the centering point is the midpoint of the film through the orbit closest to it.

Superior orbital fissure (PA). Landmarks are the forehead and nose in contact with the film; the centering point is the inferior margin of the orbits.

Mastoid process. Landmarks are the auricles of the ear (anterior) and the protruding mastoid tip; the centering (tangential) point is the anterior border of the mastoid process.

Nasal bone. Landmark is the nose and glabelloalveolar (axial view) line; the centering point is along the glabelloalveolar line and at right angles to the film.

Zygomatic arches (Fuch's position). Landmark is the zygion; the centering point is the zygion.

How is the tube shift in stereoscopic radiography determined?

The focal film distance generally determines the amount of tube shift in stereoscopic radiography. According to a rule of thumb, the tube shift should be one tenth of the focal-film distance.

In looking for suspected foreign bodies in the eye is it preferable to use screens or cardboard holders?

Since speed is important in examination of the eye to eliminate motion, screens are preferable. However, some radiologists prefer cardboard holders to secure better detail and to eliminate any possible artifact that might be produced by a foreign body in the cassette.

Define intraoral and extraoral radiography.

Intraoral radiography is a procedure concerned with the radiographic examination of the teeth that is made by placing the films within the mouth.

Extraoral radiography is a procedure concerned with the radiographic examination of the teeth that is made by placing the film outside the mouth.

Discuss the Sweet eye localizer used in radiography of a foreign body in the eye.

The Sweet eye localizer, an apparatus used to locate foreign bodies in the eye, consists of an upright column supported by a base and an extendable bar ending in two prongs—one of which has a small cone and the other a small ball. This extendable bar is raised on the upright column until the ball is level with the pupil of the eye when the head is in the true lateral position. The ball is then positioned toward the patient's eyelid until a slight depression is made. A spring is then released, and the ball retracts 1 cm. An exposure is made in this position; the film is changed, and the tube is shifted and angled sufficiently toward the head to separate the projected image of the ball and cone (15 to 25 degrees), and a second radiograph is made.

Name the two body cavities and their contents.

The two cavities are the posterior (dorsal) cavity and the anterior (ventral) cavity. The dorsal cavity contains the vertebral column, which houses the spinal cord and the cranial portion for the brain. The anterior cavity is divided into the thoracic and abdominal portions, with the pelvic cavity belonging to the lower abdominal portion.

The thoracic cavity contains the lungs, esophagus, trachea, pleural membranes, heart and great vessels, and pericardium. The abdominal cavity contains the peritonium, liver, gallbladder, pancreas, spleen, stomach and intestines, kidneys, and ureters. The rectum, urinary bladder, and parts of the reproductive organs are located in the pelvic cavity.

Name the regions of the abdomen.

The nine regions of division for the abdomen are the right hypochondriac, epigastric, left hypochondriac, right lumbar, umbilical, left lumbar, right iliac, hypogastric, and left iliac.

Name and describe the major classifications of body habitus.

The four major classifications of body habitus are the hypersthenic, sthenic, asthenic, and hyposthenic.

The hypersthenic type of body represents about 5 percent of all persons. The body is of massive build with a broad chest. The thoracic cavity is short, resulting in the ribs being almost horizontal. The lungs are short at the apices and broad at the bases. The stomach and gallbladder are high and lie almost horizontal.

The sthenic type comprises about 50 percent of all people and is a modification of the hypersthenic. The stomach lies in a normal position, and the gallbladder usually can be found under the eleventh rib.

The asthenic type includes about 10 percent of the subjects. The body is extremely slender. The chest is narrow and shallow, with the ribs sloped downward. The apices are broad, and the bases tend to be narrow. The stomach and gallbladder are low and near the midline.

The hyposthenic type includes about 35 percent of the subjects. This body habitus is a modification of the asthenic type but leans more toward the sthenic type of individual.

What views comprise the examination of the chest?

The views of the chest might include posteroanterior, anteroposterior, right and left laterals, right and left anterior obliques, right and left posterior obliques, right and left lateral decubitus, and special lordotic positions for the apices.

In radiography of the chest in the postero-anterior position, why are the shoulders rotated forward?

In the posteroanterior projection of the chest the scapulae are superimposed upon the lung fields. The simple act of rolling the shoulders forward pulls them to the lateral aspect of the chest wall, thus removing them from the lung field.

In what view would calcification of the abdominal aorta be visualized best?

The patient is positioned to lie in the lateral recumbent position on the table with knees flexed. The body is positioned so that the abdomen is centered to the midline of the table. The film is centered so that the iliac crest lies in the lower third of the cassette. The central ray is directed to the center of the film. Care in technique should be observed so that the exposure is not too heavy and does not tend to burn the cavity contents out.

What is abdominal pneumoradiography?

Abdominal pneumoradiography is the procedure of radiographic examination of the abdominal and pelvic organs by means of some gaseous contrast medium.

What is cholegraphy?

Cholegraphy is the radiologic examination of the biliary tract by means of a contrast medium administered by mouth, by intravenous injection, or by direct introduction into the bile ducts.

Through the many years of radiologic examination of the gallbladder and biliary ducts, there have been many contrast materials utilized. List those that you remember in order of sequence.

1924-1925	Tetrabromophenolphthalein
	Tetraiodophenolphthalein
1940	Priodex
1944	Monophen
1949	Telepaque
1952	Teridex
1952-1953	Biligrafinforte
	Cholografin
1956	Duografin
	Cholografin methylglucamine
1960	Biloptin
	Orografin
1962	Bilopaque

In radiography of the gallbladder why would the patient be instructed to eat a fatty meal the morning prior to the examination and instructed not to eat any food after taking the contrast material?

The patient may be instructed to eat a meal consisting of fatty foods prior to the examination of the gallbladder to empty the gallbladder of bile in preparation for receiving the contrast material. It has been stated that a better concentration of dye is present within the previously emptied gallbladder.

The patient is instructed not to eat any food after orally taking the contrast material to restrain the gallbladder from emptying the opaque material prior to radiography. Water may be taken in small quantities. Some instructions allow tea and coffee without the cream.

Give the rule of thumb for positioning the patients of various body habitus.

By and large, by remembering the positions of the various organs within the body habitus, the technologist will position more accurately. In the hypersthenic type of individual the gallbladder usually lies under the eighth rib, in the horizontal position and in the lateral aspect of the abdominal cavity. In the sthenic type individual the gallbladder lies in the midline of the median plane and lateral aspect of the abdominal cavity under the eleventh rib. In the asthenic individual the gallbladder may lie in the lower abdominal cavity in the region of the pelvis and close to the median plane.

What views may be taken in a gallbladder examination?

The gallbladder examination may consist of an anteroposterior (scout), posteroanterior oblique, posteroanterior oblique crest, and right lateral decubitus views. In some instances fluoroscopic spot films may be taken. If necessary, laminographic cuts may be ordered.

The gastrointestinal series would include what examinations?

The routine gastrointestinal series would include the following:

A scout film of the abdomen would be taken to check on the cleaning procedure of the patient. It is used to check the liver, spleen, kidneys, and general cleanliness of the patient. The detection of visual pathology is checked at this time.

The patient is then fluoroscoped with the injection of some contrast material, usually barium sulfate. Radiographic and fluoroscopic studies of the esophagus, stomach, and duodenum are then taken.

A small bowel study is sometimes requested, with films of the abdomen taken at frequent intervals to ascertain the passage of the barium.

Discuss the preparation of the patient for a gastrointestinal series.

Since good delineation of the gastrointestinal tract depends upon having the patient properly prepared, it is important that the stomach be empty and the colon free from gas and feces. Usually a cathartic is prescribed the evening before and may be followed by a cleaning enema in the evening and another in the early morning following the cathartic action. All food and water are withheld from midnight of the evening before the examination. Some preparations consist of placing the patient on a low-residue diet 2 or 3 days prior to the examination to prevent gas formation in the intestines.

In examination of the small bowel the patient may be held within the radiology department for further films. In the event that the patient is allowed to return to the ward before completion of the gastrointestinal studies, he should be instructed not to eat or drink anything until allowed to do so. He should be instructed when to return to the department for further studies.

When the examination is completed, the patient should be advised to drink water freely to prevent impaction of the barium within the colon. When indicated, a cathartic may be given.

How should barium sulfate be mixed for study of the gastrointestinal tract?

The formula using barium sulfate that has proved successful in the examination of the gastrointestinal tract is to have the solution contain equal parts of barium and water by volume. The consistency should be that of heavy cream. The ingredients should be thoroughly mixed, preferably with an electric mixer. There is a tendency on the part of some radiology departments to add a flavoring substance to the barium preparation. A preparation of carboxymethylcellulose, 5 percent solution, may be added to the solution for better adherence to the mucosal wall.

What procedure would you follow to radiograph the esophagus?

The patient is given the barium sulfate in the form of either paste or solution. With paste the patient takes a mouthful and chews it to a consistency for easy swallowing. To outline the esophagus in a preliminary manner several mouthfuls are consumed before the radiograph is taken.

To demonstrate esophageal varices the patient receives a mouthful of barium solution, exhales to the fullest extent, and swallows the barium. The breath is held in exhalation during the exposure. Another method is to take a mouthful of barium and inhale fully. While holding the breath in inspiration, the barium is swallowed, and the patient is instructed to perform the Valsalva maneuver.

To demonstrate the entire esophagus the patient is instructed to drink a creamy mixture of barium through a straw continuously during the exposure of the film.

What is the Valsalva maneuver?

In the true Valsalva maneuver the patient takes in a deep breath and, while holding that breath, bears down as if to move his bowels. This maneuver forces the air against the closed glottis and increases the intrathoracic and intra-abdominal pressure.

In the modified Valsalva maneuver the patient is asked to pinch his nose tightly and to hold his mouth closed. While doing this, he is asked to attempt to blow through his nose.

What is spot filming?

Spot-film radiography is a procedure used when attention is to be focused on a particular area of a larger anatomic part. Such a procedure is quite common in gastrointestinal work or in myelography in which, during fluoroscopy, a site of pathology may become visible, and the fluoroscopist will immediately make spot films of that particular area, using the same tube employed during fluoroscopy.

Why are oblique views made in radiographic examinations of the stomach?

Oblique views are made for three reasons. First, these views delineate different portions of the stomach wall in profile. Second, because of the superimposition of the spine over the stomach in the posteroanterior position, it is necessary to rotate the patient. Third, oblique views are used to demonstrate the duodenal cap.

Describe the nature and use of barium sulfate in radiography.

Barium sulfate is a radiopaque preparation derived from one of the natural salts of barium. This preparation is used in radiography for the examination of portions of the gastrointestinal system. Barium sulfate fills or outlines the part being examined and produces a shadow on the fluoroscopic screen or film.

What is the purpose of a gastrointestinal motility series?

The gastrointestinal motility series is performed to demonstrate the peristaltic function of the digestive tract and to detect pathology concerned with the passage of barium or other contrast material.

What is the Chassard-Lapine position in radiography of the colon, and what is its purpose?

The Chassard-Lapine position is used to demonstrate the rectum, rectosigmoid junction, and sigmoid. It allows the sigmoid to become uncoiled and projected free from overlapping.

The patient is seated on the side of the table with the buttocks placed in the midline of the table. The thighs are abducted as far as possible. The patient is asked to lean forward as far as possible and to grasp his ankles for support. The film is centered to the median plane, and the central ray is directed perpendicular to the film through the lumbosacral region at the level of the greater trochanters.

What is intravenous radiography?

Intravenous radiography is a procedure in which films are made after an opaque medium has been injected into a vein. Usually, such a procedure is followed in examinations of the kidneys, venous systems, and hepatic and common ducts.

What do you understand retrograde pyelography to be?

Retrograde pyelography is a radiographic procedure for examination of the kidneys and urinary tract. This procedure is accomplished by inserting catheters into the ureters through which an opaque medium is injected. A film or films are made of the kidneys and/or ureters.

What positions would you use to demonstrate kidney stones?

Kidney stones may be visualized with the patient in the anteroposterior, lateral, either or both obliques (depending upon which kidney is involved), and upright positions. In some instances the patient may be taken in the posteroanterior position.

What preparation would you suggest for intravenous pyelography?

To properly prepare a patient for intravenous pyelography, the patient may be placed on a low-residue diet for 2 or 3 days prior to scheduling the examination. On the day prior to the examination a cathartic is given in the evening, and all foods and fluids are withheld after the light evening meal. A cleansing enema is given the evening before and the morning of the examination.

What are the various methods used to demonstrate the genitourinary system?

In radiography of the genitourinary system, an examination may include a scout film in which no contrast medium is used. Intravenous pyelography, in which a contrast medium is injected into the vein and secreted by the kidneys, and retrograde pyelography, in which a contrast medium is instilled into the kidneys through a catheter, are other methods of examining the genitourinary system. Cystography is a procedure in which contrast material is instilled into the urinary bladder through a catheter and radiographs are taken.

What is body-section radiography?

Body-section radiography is a technique in which, with special equipment, a radiograph of some predetermined level in the body is taken. This is done by moving the x-ray tube and film in opposing directions about a fulcrum that is set at a preselected level. Since the fulcrum level will remain stationary during the exposure, the relating body area or level will be in sharp focus, while levels above and below the fulcrum point will be out of focus and will be blurred.

What is myelography?

Myelography is an x-ray procedure in which a small amount of spinal fluid is first removed by spinal tap and replaced with an opaque medium. Under fluoroscopic control and by angulating the table, this opaque medium is manipulated through the spinal canal. By this means complete or partial obstruction and deviations from normal may be detected. Spot films are often an integral part of this examination.

What is ventriculography?

Ventriculography is a method of radiographically examining the ventricular system of the brain as well as the brain tissue itself. Ventriculography may be, and usually is, an operating room procedure. A burr hole is made on each side of the mid-sagittal plane in line with the occipital horns of the lateral ventricles. Needles are inserted through these holes into the lateral ventricles. Air or gas is injected into the ventricles and a similar amount of fluid removed. When a satisfactory exchange of gas and fluid is complete, the needles are removed and the openings closed. The degree of filling and pathology are demonstrated because the air in the ventricles is less dense than the surrounding skull area. A series of skull radiographs is taken with the patient in a number of positions.

What is cerebral angiography?

Cerebral angiography is a method of radiographically examining the circulatory system of the brain for the localization and identification of intracranial lesions. In this procedure an aqueous opaque medium is injected, under pressure, into the carotid artery. Radiographs are made serially and in rapid succession to record the flow of this opaque medium through the circulatory system. Usually, this procedure calls for some method of rapid film changing, fractional second exposures and from four to twelve or more radiographs per second.

What is cardioangiography?

Cardioangiography is a method of radiographically examining the circulatory system of the heart and great vessels. In this procedure an aqueous opaque solution is injected into the chambers of the heart or into the brachial artery. Radiographs are made serially and in rapid succession to record the progression of the opaque medium through the circulatory system. This examination calls for a method of rapid film changing, fractional second exposures, and a number of exposures, as many as twelve per second.

What is cholangiography?

Cholangiography is a method of radiographically examining the bile ducts after the instillation of opaque medium. This examination is usually postoperative and is accomplished by direct instillation of the opaque medium (per T tube) into the ducts or by an intravenous injection of the opaque medium into the circulatory system of the patient.

What is xeroradiography?

Xeroradiography is a method of performing radiographic examinations making use of conventional x-ray generating equipment but substituting a selenium-coated plate for the silver bromide emulsion film. Conventional processing procedures are replaced in favor of a so-called dry-processing method. In use the selenium-coated plate is charged electrically, the plate is positioned beneath the patient, and the exposure is made. The exposure to radiation discharges the plate in the area covered by the anatomic part in proportion to its thickness and opacity. The plate is then placed in a special unit and sprayed with a fine powder. This in turn makes the patient's radiographic image visible. The selenium-coated plate can be recharged and reexposed a number of times, and thus it is not rendered useless for further application as a recording medium.

What does image-intensification mean?

Image-intensification is a system for electrically intensifying the low light emission level of a fluoroscopic screen. Intensification can reach a point at which the eye's rod and cone perceptors are both stimulated, thus resulting in much better visual acuity. With the usual fluoroscopic screen only rod vision is possible, unless the milliamperage is excessively increased. Image-intensification systems pick up the light from a regular fluoroscopic screen on a photoemission surface, electronically amplify it, and then convert it back to a higher light level. Another image-intensification method is to bombard a photoconductor with radiation to produce a direct electric signal, thus eliminating the fluoroscopic screen. The electric signal is then amplified and cast onto a viewing medium.

Name the radiographic examinations used to demonstrate the internal structures of the cranium.

To demonstrate the internal structures of the cranium the following radiographic examinations may be used:
1. Routine skull series
2. Special views for particular anatomic parts
3. Cerebral angiography
4. Ventriculography
5. Pneumoencephalography
6. Body section radiography

If a patient is referred to the radiology department with fluid in the chest, what positions should be taken?

To show fluid in the lungs the technologist may take an upright posteroanterior and lateral chest film. If unable to do the posteroanterior view, the anteroposterior view will suffice. Right and left lateral decubitus films may also be taken.

What radiographic examination should be associated with ventriculography?

Ventriculography is associated with the radiographic examination of the ventricular system of the brain. The examination is performed by a direct puncture into the lateral ventricle. The cerebrospinal fluid is removed and replaced with air. Radiographic exposures are taken at various intervals to demonstrate the flow and position of the air and to outline the ventricles.

How does pneumoencephalography differ from ventriculography?

Pneumoencephalography is a study of the brain tissue as well as the ventricles of the brain. In this examination the spinal fluid is removed by means of a spinal puncture and is replaced by air. The air, being lighter than the fluid, flows into and outlines the ventricles. The air is less dense than the brain tissue, and thus the tissue is demonstrated.

What is meant by immobilization, and how is it accomplished?

Immobilization is the method of minimizing motion on the part of the patient. The following are various methods of accomplishing this:
1. The cloth immobilizing band is attached to castings and arranged so that it can be moved the entire length of the x-ray table. It is adjusted by means of a ratchet system. Care must be used with this device to prevent patient rotation in the direction of the winding mechanism.
2. Head clamps are utilized in the radiographic examination of the skull and sinuses.
3. Sandbags are utilized in the radiography of extremities.
4. Many commercial immobilization devices that use special taping mechanisms are available.
5. Special children's immobilization devices can be secured from commercial companies.

9 SPECIAL PROCEDURES

Since the advent of radiology as a profession, many changes have taken place. Not the least of these has been the perfection of procedures to visualize organs within the body that previously had been hidden. All the technologic advances in equipment design and contrast materials that may be safely injected have played an important part. These new procedures have been labeled as special procedures. This denotes that they are not routinely performed but require the addition of some foreign material to cause them to become visible. The newer equipment now obtainable allows the visualization and recording of areas and procedures that were previously not available.

The injection of any material foreign to the system carries with it a certain risk, and every precaution should be exercised to assure the administration of the proper and correct material in accurate amounts. Various names have been given to different procedures, but they usually denote the area under examination.

Angiocardiography is a procedure designed to do what?

Angiocardiography demonstrates the internal anatomy of the heart and great vessels.

The contrast medium is usually delivered in angiocardiography by what method?

When doing angiocardiography, the injections are usually done by simultaneous injection into the veins of both arms.

If, when doing a venous angiocardiogram, the left ventricle is shown to opacify before the pulmonary arteries, what does this indicate?

This is indicative of an abnormal pathway of blood flow from the right side to the left side of the heart.

If selective right ventricular angiocardiography is done, what would be the sequence of opacification of the structures visualized?

In right ventricular angiocardiography the structures would opacify in the following sequence: right ventricle, pulmonary arteries and veins, left atrium, left ventricle, and aorta.

The flow of blood or contrast medium through the heart is very rapid, and films for permanent records must be made. What recording system is generally used?

A rapid film changer is normally used, preferably one that can operate at fractions of a second. To demonstrate the four chambers of the heart in an adult, the usual time of circulation is between ten and fifteen seconds.

When may a catheter be introduced

through a femoral artery in doing ventricular angiocardiography?

When selective angiocardiography of the ventricular system is required, a catheter may be introduced through a femoral artery.

What technique is used principally for arteriography?

The Seldinger technique is used principally for arteriography.

In doing an abdominal aortogram which arteries would be visualized?

The arteries visualized would be the renal, inferior mesenteric, inferior phrenic, and celiac.

When should a percutaneous transfemoral arteriogram not be done?

This examination should not be done when there is an occlusion of the lower abdominal aorta.

For what purpose is aortography performed?

When there are suspected occlusions or other symptoms to indicate trouble with the major arteries of the trunk, aortography is performed.

What is the oldest and most widely used method of aortography?

Direct puncture of the abdominal aorta is the oldest and most widely used method.

When performing aortography, the renal arteries are visualized arising from where?

The renal arteries arise from the aorta below the superior mesenteric and above the inferior mesenteric.

Who was the first person to perform translumbar aortography?

Dos Santos was the first person to perform translumbar aortography.

What examination is performed for the detection of enlarged lymph nodes in the abdomen?

To detect enlarged lymph nodes in the abdomen, inferior vena cavography would be performed.

The thoracic duct, considered to be the main lymph duct of the body, originating at the cisterna chyli on the abdomen, serves what function?

The thoracic duct conveys lymph from the lymph nodes to the subclavian veins. It receives lymph from all parts of the body except the right side of the head, neck, thorax, and right upper extremity.

To study the blood vessels in the lungs, what methods may be used?

Several methods may be used—intravenous angiography, passage of a catheter to the pulmonary artery with injection, passage of a catheter to the superior vena cava with injection, or bronchial arteriography.

If a leaking mitral valve is suspected and a ventricular angiocardiogram is to be done, what would be the sequence of opacification of structures?

If a patient has a leaking mitral valve, the left ventricle, left atrium, and aorta respectively would opacify when a left ventricular angiocardiogram was done.

What examinations are performed for visualization of the kidneys?

Intravenous pyelograms, retrograde pyelograms, nephrotomography, renal arteriography, and cyst puncture are performed for kidney visualization.

Which of the following examinations is performed by an intravenous injection of contrast material: retrograde pyelography, cystourethrography, retroperitoneal air insufflation, nephrotomography, or renal arteriography?

Of the examinations listed nephrotomography is performed by intravenous injection.

Is fluoroscopy used when examining the kidneys?

Normally, for most examinations of the kidneys, fluoroscopy is not used, but when doing a cyst puncture it is important that it be performed under fluoroscopic control.

For what purpose is a cholangiogram done during surgery?

A cholangiogram is usually done to demonstrate the major biliary ducts as being free from obstructions.

For what is percutaneous transhepatic cholangiography usually performed?

Percutaneous transhepatic cholangiography is performed for visualization of the bile duct to determine whether an obstruction is present.

Why is celiac angiography performed?

Celiac angiography is usually performed to demonstrate the vessels of the liver, spleen, stomach, and pancreas.

What is probably the most accurate way to demonstrate esophageal varices?

Splenoportography is probably the most accurate demonstration of esophageal varices.

To check for gross anatomy of the female reproductive organs, what examination is performed?

Pelvic pneumography is probably the most effective examination, and it involves the use of nitrous oxide, which is both safe and effective, as a medium.

What is pelvimetry?

Pelvimetry is a radiographic technique that allows measurement of the dimensions of the pelvis to determine whether or not the pelvis is large enough for the fetus to pass through and be born in a normal manner.

What is hysterosalpingography?

Hysterosalpingography is the opacification of the lumen of the uterus and fallopian tubes by injection of an oily contrast material.

Which contrast material is normally used in doing hysterosalpingography?

The oily contrast material used is Salpix.

What are the procedures that may be used for diagnosing placenta praevia?

Any of these procedures—amniography, uterine arteriography, and isotopic localization—may be done for diagnosing placenta praevia.

What is carotid arteriography?

Carotid arteriography is the study of the arteries of the brain by injection of contrast material into the carotid artery. Injection is usually made into the common carotid artery.

How many arteries supply the brain?

Four arteries—two on each side—supply the brain. They are the carotid and vertebral arteries.

The carotid artery has several branches. Which branch lies near the midline?

The branch of the carotid artery lying near the midline is the anterior cerebral artery.

What is pneumoencephalography?

Pneumoencephalography is the procedure in which spinal fluid is taken from the body and replaced with air or a gas. A needle is inserted into the spinal canal, and spinal fluid is withdrawn in small amounts, with air being injected.

In what position is the patient during the beginning of pneumoencephalography?

The patient is usually seated with his head flexed forward.

Which is the first ventricle to fill during pneumoencephalography?

The first ventricle to fill is the fourth.

What views are usually taken during pneumoencephalography?

Erect PA, lateral, prone PA, and lateral, supine AP; "brow up" and prone "brow down"; and a Towne's position are usually taken during pneumoencephalography.

What is myelography?

Myelography is the study of the spinal canal by the injection of an oily substance into the canal. It is usually performed under fluoroscopic control with films taken of any abnormalities.

What contrast agent is usually used to outline the spinal cord and nerve roots?

In the United States the agent generally used is Pantopaque.

What is arthrography?

Arthrography is the procedure used for demonstration of the joint spaces and the structure within them.

What is a diskogram?

A diskogram is the examination of the disk space between the vertebrae and is performed by the insertion of a needle into the disk with the injection of a contrast material. It demonstrates a rupture if one is present.

What is azygography?

Azygography is a procedure usually performed by injecting contrast material into a rib.

Of what advantage are stereo films?

Stereo films are advantageous because they help to localize structures by providing a three-dimensional effect.

If arterial hemorrhage occurs after an arterial puncture, what should the technician do until the doctor arrives?

The technician should apply pressure upon the artery.

What are the major differences between encephalography and ventriculography?

Encephalography is the radiographic examination of the brain after replacement of the cerebrospinal fluid with air introduced by a lumbar puncture, whereas ventriculography is a system that demonstrates the ventricles by drilling small holes into the cranial vault and insterting needles directly into the ventricles.

What is bronchography?

Bronchography is the examination of the bronchi and bronchioles by the injection of a contrast medium. If pathology is suspected, this side is filled first and films taken before the opposite side is opacified.

What is kymography?

Kymography is a system for recording on film the motions of the various organs, particularly the heart and great vessels.

What is cystography?

The study of the bladder by injection of a contrast medium through a catheter is known as cystography.

What is sialography?

Sialography is the study of the parotid and submaxillary glands. A cannula is inserted into the ducts and a contrast medium injected.

When is lymphangiography performed?

When it is necessary to demonstrate the lymph nodes and potency of the vessels to determine the involvement of pathology, a lymphangiography is performed.

When performing inferior vena cavography, what structures are visualized?

This examination demonstrates the inferior vena cava, retroperitoneal space, kidneys, ureters, and bladder.

10 DARKROOM

What is meant by a darkroom?

A darkroom is a room devoid of all white light in which the processing cycle of the exposed x-ray film may take place. Unlike its name, the room is not entirely dark but has illumination of safe density to allow technicians to perform their work accurately and safely. The darkroom may be used for other incidentals necessary to the efficient operation of the department, for example, the loading and unloading of cassettes.

What is the processing cycle?

The processing cycle consists of the various procedures that produce a visible image on an exposed film. These procedures are developing, rinsing, fixing, washing, and drying.

What source of illumination may be used in the darkroom?

The source of illumination in the darkroom is a safelight, which is constructed so that it will not fog an x-ray film within a reasonable time of exposure to it.

What safelight in the darkroom is considered safe?

A safelight that utilizes a Wratten 6B filter and uses a bulb of correct wattage designed for use in the safelight is safe for a nominal time interval.

Why is using the correct wattage so important?

To use or replace a bulb with one of lower wattage in the safelight does no damage at all, except to cut down the overall darkroom illumination.

To use or replace a bulb with one of higher wattage has disadvantages. The first disadvantage is that the increased illumination from the higher wattage cuts down on the safe time that a film may be exposed to it before becoming fogged. Second, the higher temperature of the bulb may cause the filter to crack.

How would the technologist test a safelight for safety?

The safelight may be tested for safety by placing an exposed film on the bench. The film is covered with a piece of cardboard so that only about 2 inches of the lower end of the film is exposed. This is left for a minute; then the cardboard is moved upward another 2 inches, and the film is exposed another minute. This procedure is repeated continuously until the whole film is exposed. It is noted that if a 10- x 12-inch film were used, the lower strip would have received five minutes of exposure, and the upper strip one minute. The film is processed and inspected. When the first signs of fogging are seen, this will indicate the time allowable for the film to be exposed to the safelight. If this allowable time is too short, the wattage of the bulb may be changed to a lower one or the safelight raised to a greater distance from the film. In either case the experiment should be repeated.

What is meant by the term "developer"?

The term "developer" indicates solutions that will convert the exposed silver bromide crystals of the photographic image on the x-ray film to a visible image. Chemically it is a reducing solution that reduces the exposed silver halide crystals to black metallic silver. It is always alkaline in nature; because it is, the gelatin swells to allow the reducing agents to attack and work on the exposed crystals. The amount of alkalinity is determined by checking its pH factor.

Name the chemicals that comprise the developing solution.

The chemicals that make up the developer are elon or metal, hydroquinone, sodium sulfite, sodium carbonate, and potassium bromide.

What specific functions do these chemicals have in the developing solution?

Elon is a developing or reducing agent that builds up detail quickly in the first half of the development period.

Hydroquinone is a developing or reducing agent that builds up contrast slowly during the development period.

Both of the previous developing agents reduce exposed silver bromide crystals in emulsion to black metallic silver constituting the image.

Sodium sulfite is a preservative that prevents rapid oxidation of the developer.

Sodium carbonate is an alkali or activator that governs reducing activities of developing agents. It provides necessary alkaline medium and swells gelatin emulsion so that reducing agents can attack exposed silver bromide crystals.

Potassium bromide is a restrainer that controls activity of reducing agents and tends to prevent fog.

What is meant by "oxidized developer," and how can be be prevented?

Oxidized developer is that which has become exhausted because of exposure to light and air as well as the action of the bromide and hydrogen ions. The speed at which oxidation occurs may be delayed by replacing the cover on the developing solutions when not in use. The cover can even be placed over the tank during development of films.

How can you test for oxidized developer?

If you suspect the developer to be oxidized, you may expose a film with a given technique: split the film in two and develop one half in a known proper developer solution and the other half in the suspected oxidized developer. The oxidized developer will be light and often will stain the film because of the oxidation. However, it is a good rule to change the solution whenever the developing time exceeds that of good developing.

What is considered to be optimum developing time?

The film and chemical manufacturers recommend five minutes at 68° F. for the optimum developing time.

What reactions do the developer chemicals have at higher or lower temperatures?

Perhaps the developer chemical most affected by changes in temperature is hydroquinone. This chemical is the most active and controls the density and contrast. However, at lower temperatures (60° F. and below) the chemical loses activity rapidly and does not produce good results. When the temperature rises, the activity becomes rapid and intense, and, as before, the result is degraded.

What is the fixing solution?

The fixing solution, known as hypo, is used to clear the unexposed and undeveloped silver halide crystals from the film, leaving only the exposed and developed silver halide crystals on the film to form the permanent image.

Name the chemicals making up the fixing, or hypo, solution.

The chemicals making up the fixing solution are sodium thiosulfate, sodium sulfite, acetic acid, and potassium alum.

What are the specific functions of the chemicals in the fixing solution?

Sodium thiosulfate is a fixing agent that dissolves unexposed silver bromide crystals but does not affect reduced metallic silver of image.

Sodium sulfite is a preservative that maintains the equilibrium of chemicals in solution.

Acetic acid is an acidifier that provides acid medium and neutralizes developer carried over in film.

Potassium alum is a hardening agent that shrinks and hardens emulsion.

What is meant by the term "fog"?

The term "fog" is used to indicate an overall increase in unwanted density of the processed film. The three types are chemical, radiation, and light.

What is meant by chemical fog?

Chemical fog is an overall increase of gray density on the x-ray film and is produced by a very strong solution, overdevelopment of the film, or old developer that has been unused. Prolonged overdevelopment will result in a discoloration (brownish appearance) on the film.

What are radiation fog and light fog?

Radiation fog is an increase in the overall density of the film, which is usually superimposed upon the original density.

It is caused by radiation striking the film either before or after exposure.

Light fog is usually seen as a blackening of the film where the light has struck it.

How can fog be prevented?

Chemical fog may be prevented by using the time-temperature method of development and correct changing periods for solutions.

Radiation fog may be prevented by proper storage of x-ray film in lead containers or at a safe distance from the radiation source.

Light fog may be prevented by sealing all avenues of light in the darkroom and using proper safelights. Warped cassettes or worn felts on cassettes should be fixed.

What does the term "shortstop" denote?

The term "shotstop" denotes a solution that will completely stop the action of the developing solution before placing the film into the fixer. The shortstop is usually a weak solution of acetic acid.

If a box of films is suspected of being fogged, how should they be tested to see if it is true?

To test for suspected fog the technologist would remove three unexposed films from the package (one from the front portion, one from the middle, and one from the rear). The unexposed films would then be processed. Visual inspection of the films would determine the extent, if any, of the fogging.

What is an artifact, and how are they prevented?

An artifact is any marking on a film that is foreign to that film. Some of them are treelike effects as a result of static electricity, finger marks, crinkles, crescent-shaped marks cause by sharp bending of film, and white spots on film because of dirty intensifying screens.

Artifacts can be prevented by careful

handling of the films and utilizing the laws of cleanliness in the department. Film benches should be grounded so that static electricity accumulated by the technologist can be dissipated.

What factors must be considered in the storage and handling of unexposed x-ray film?

The following factors must be considered:
1. Films begin to age upon manufacture. To ensure proper usage the film manufacturers stamp upon each film box an expiration date. Care should be taken to use the older films first.
2. Films should be stored in a cool and dry area. Heat and moisture have adverse effects upon the emulsion. To help prevent this, the film manufacturers have wrapped the film in moisture-sealed packages.
3. Films should be stored in areas that are free from radiation sources. They should be shielded, if necessary. However, distance is a good protective device.
4. Films are sensitive to light and therefore should be opened only in proper darkrooms.

Explain the construction of x-ray film.

Modern x-ray film is manufactured utilizing a base and an emulsion upon the base. The base consists of a sheet of cellulose acetate or polyester, about 0.0008 inch thick. Film manufacturers usually tint the base to a desired color. The base is nonexplosive.

The emulsion consists of silver bromide crystals suspended in a gelatinous solution. This mixture is heated to a temperature of 50° to 80° C. for purposes of increasing the sensitivity of the emulsion. This process is termed "digestion." The emulsion is then coated on both sides of the base. The emulsion layer is about 0.0001 inch thick. The film is then allowed to cool and age until it is ready to be cut

into the proper sizes. The emulsion has certain sensitivity and latitude characteristics built into it by the film manufacturer. The speed/sensitivity of the film concerns the ability of the film to respond to x-rays and light. Film latitude deals with the ability of the emulsion to record tonal differences when exposed to radiation. It also allows for errors in radiographic technique.

What types of film for medical radiography are in use today?

Primarily, two types of film are in use today. They are screen film and nonscreen film.

Screen film is perhaps more widely used than nonscreen film. It is sensitive to the blue light spectrum given off by the intensifying screens and also to direct exposure of x-rays.

Nonscreen film cannot be used in conjunction with cassettes and screens. The thicker emulsion of the film makes it impervious to penetration by light. Nonscreen film is dependent upon direct exposure of the x-ray beam. Because of its thicker emulsion and increase in silver bromide crystals, the film is about four times faster than screen film used in a cardboard holder.

Before the introduction of cellulose acetate films, the x-ray image was recorded on what medium?

Prior to cellulose acetate base films, x-ray images were recorded on glass plates coated with an emulsion sensitive to light. These plates had disadvantages in that there was always the danger of breakage, awkwardness in processing (cut hands and fingers from broken edges of the plate), and the problem of filing.

Explain the difference between screen film and nonscreen film.

1. Nonscreen film has a thicker coating of emulsion than the screen film.
2. Nonscreen film is faster than screen film because of its thicker coating of

emulsion and greater amount of silver bromide crystals.

3. Under compatible conditions the non-screen film will produce shorter scales of contrast than will screen film.
4. In the hand processing cycle the non-screen film requires about two minutes more of development time than does the screen film.
5. The nonscreen film does not fix as rapidly as does the screen film.

What is meant by film speed?

The speed of the film is the ability of the film emulsion to react to x-rays or light in short exposure periods and to produce radiographs of suitable densities.

What is film latitude?

To the technologist latitude has meant the built-in margin of error for any given technique that will not affect too visibly the finished radiograph. However, latitude also means the ability of the film emulsion to record an image in either long- or short-scale contrast.

How are radiographic films packaged?

Radiographic films are packaged in various ways, from boxes of 25- to 1,000-sheet thrift packs. Some boxes are paper interleaved, whereas the larger packaged films do not have the paper. The film manufacturer determines the best means of packaging the film.

What is meant by film expiration date, and why is it important?

The film expiration date is placed upon each box of film by the manufacturer to denote the time that the film will lose its useful range in radiography.

To prevent loss of film the technologist should always use the film with the shortest remaining expiration date. When placing new film with longer expiration dates in storage, care should be taken to place in the front those with the shorter expiration dates.

What is photoradiographic film?

Photoradiographic film is film that is coated only on one side and is used in mass chest survey work to record the patient image from a fluoroscopic screen.

What is dosimeter film?

Dosimeter film is manufactured to record high-energy radiation dosage. It is packaged in dental-size packets that may contain different types of film to record various dosage ranges.

What is meant by duplicating film?

Duplicating film is a special, single-coated film used to produce a direct positive copy of a finished radiograph.

What is the polaroid radiographic film?

The polaroid radiographic film is a special film that will develop as a paper-based translucency print. It is used with a special cassette and developed by means of a special roller development machine. The paper-based print, known as 3,000×, requires ten seconds to process. Type TLX translucency film requires forty-five seconds to develop.

How are dental films classified?

Dental films are classified as periapical, occlusal, and interproximal.

What would you consider the term "monopack" to mean when referring to x-ray film?

The term "monopack," when referring to x-ray film, denotes the packaging conditions of the x-ray film. Each film is packaged in an individual lightproof envelope and is used as if the film were in a cardboard holder.

What is meant by the latent image?

The x-ray film is coated on both sides with an emulsion containing silver bromide crystals. Whereas the formation of the latent image is a chemical process, it may be described simply as follows: The emulsion on the film is struck by radiation or light, and a chemical change takes place in proportion to the amount of radiation or light absorbed by the silver bromide crystals in the emulsion. If an object is placed between the source of radiation and the film, the absorbing qualities of the object will diminish the radiation reaching the film. The quality of radiation reaching the film will vary. The chemical reaction of these various qualities upon the silver bromide crystals will produce an image with varying radiographic densities. Thus the latent image may be described as that image formed on the film by radiation or light prior to development.

What is meant by postexposure fog when referring to an x-ray film?

Postexposure fog usually occurs in the darkroom and is often the result of exposure to a safelight of higher-than-necessary wattage. The technologist must remember that previously exposed radiographic films are eight times more sensitive to fog than unexposed films.

What are some conditions for good darkroom planning?

1. The term "darkroom" may be a misnomer in this day and age since we do not utilize darkrooms completely when developing our radiographic film. However, the darkroom should exclude all white light. This means that the doors and outlets must be lightproof and all safelight filters must be in good condition.

2. Whenever possible, the darkroom should be centrally located with relation to the radiographic rooms. The theory has recently been put forth that every four radiographic rooms should be serviced by one darkroom for more efficient operation.

3. A method of entrance into the darkroom should be constructed with either the maze or labyrinth type or the interlocking type of doors. This would tend to eliminate the accidental opening of the darkroom door while films are being processed.

4. The size of the darkroom will vary with the conditions of operation and the size of the department. One must realize that it should be adequate to house all the necessary equipment for good darkroom operation.

5. A good darkroom will be properly illuminated. Various types of lighting should be available within the darkroom area. They are proper safelight, a view box by which to inspect the finished radiograph, and overhead or general illumination to use when cleaning the darkroom.

6. A proper method of ventilation to aid in the exchange of air within the darkroom should be included.

Why is good ventilation necessary in the darkroom?

Good ventilation or exchange of air is necessary to promote efficient operation by darkroom personnel. It removes odors and stale air and replaces them with fresh air, which is essential to good health practices. The best method of ventilation is air conditioning.

What is meant by film processing?

Film processing is the conversion of the latent image to a visible image and the preservation of that image as a permanent record. The processing cycle consists of developing, rinsing, fixing, washing, and drying.

What is meant by time-temperature development?

Perhaps the most important factors of the development cycle are time and temperature. Time refers to the length of stay in the developing solution and temperature the degree of hotness or coldness of the solution. As the temperature of the solution increases, the time of the development decreases. Conversely, as the temperature decreases, the development time increases.

What is sight developing?

Sight developing is the inspection of the film at various intervals of time during the development process to determine the correct density factor or, more often, to save a film that has been improperly exposed. Visual inspection is accomplished by utilizing the developing tank safelight.

What is the purpose of agitation during the development cycle?

When initially placed into the developer, the film should be agitated to dislodge any air bubbles that may be clinging to the film.

Agitation of the film should be performed periodically to replace exhausted developer solution in contact with the film with fresh solution.

Agitation also provides uniform development for the film.

What is hypo neutralizer?

Hypo neutralizer is a solution used between the fixing solution and the final washing cycle to reduce the washing time of the films. Properly fixed films, when immersed in this solution, require only five minutes of washing time. With adequate drying facilities this may speed the efficiency of the darkroom, but without adequate drying facilities it is a waste.

What is a wetting agent, and why is it used?

The wetting agent is a solution used at the completion of the washing cycle to reduce the surface tension of the water on the film and thus allow it to drain more rapidly. It helps prevent the formation of water spots on the film.

What causes processed radiographic films to "yellow" after storage for a period of time?

Processed radiographic films will discolor after a period of time in storage because of a chemical reaction caused by the retention of fixing solutions within the film as the result of improper washing cycle. It may also occur when films have not been properly fixed.

What is meant by image reversal, and how is it caused?

Image reversal is the changing of the radiographic image from the positive to the negative. The blacks appear as whites and the whites as blacks. This may occur when the overhead white light is momentarily turned on during the development cycle.

What does the term "black metallic silver" mean?

Black metallic silver occurs after the exposure of a radiographic film to radiation and the consequent change of the exposed silver bromide crystals in the latent image to the visible black metallic in the development cycle.

What is considered to be the normal fixing time of a radiograph?

The normal fixing time of a radiograph is considered to be twice the clearing time. As the fixing solution becomes exhausted, the fixing time will increase. Therefore, if the clearing time of a film is one minute, the fixing time will be two minutes.

What is fog?

Fog is a supplemental density that covers the radiographic film. It is caused by secondary radiation, chemical fog, and light fog.

Secondary radiation is scattered rays of radiation that are radiographically effective and cause a fairly uniform deposit of silver over the entire image. It is characterized by a dull gray appearance on the film and the absence of good visible detail.

Chemical fog is caused during the development cycle and is the result of overdevelopment or development at extremely high temperatures. It also can be caused by exhausted developing solutions. It usually has the appearance of a brown stain.

Light fog occurs when the light (white) in the darkroom is turned on, the safelight has cracked glass, the safelight bulb wattage is too high, the exposed film is left under the safelight too long, or the darkroom is not light tight. It has the appearance of overall blackening of the film.

What is automatic processing?

Automatic processing is the development of the exposed radiographic films by means of a machine that continually feeds the film from one solution to another and through the drying cycle, emerging as a finished radiograph. Originally the automatic processing was regulated to seven minutes; it has now been reduced to ninety seconds in many instances but may be regulated to three and one-half minutes.

Are there advantages to having automatic processing?

Yes, the following are advantages to automatic film processing:
1. It eliminates the need for reading wet films to get an immediate reading.
2. It gives uniform processing.
3. It improves the radiographic technique in the radiology department.
4. It improves patient care by efficiency in operation.
5. It facilitates expansion of the departmental work load.

What are some recommended developing temperatures of automatic processing?

Some of the developing temperatures of automatic processing are as follows:
$$80° \text{ to } 84° \text{ F.—7 minutes}$$
$$90° \text{ F.—3½ minutes}$$
$$90° \text{ to } 103° \text{ F.—90 seconds}$$

The manufacturer of automatic processors recommends specific ways of feeding various sizes of film. What are they?

Film that is 10 × 12 inches or larger should be placed with the larger side entering the machine, that is, 17 inches for a 14 × 17 inch. Film sizes smaller than 10 × 12 inches should be placed with the smaller side preceding. In this manner two films may be processed simultaneously.

What is meant by the exhaustion of the chemical solutions?

Exhaustion of the chemical solutions is the inability of the chemicals to react in their proper way because of the rate of oxidation of the solution, the number of films processed, and the presence of contamination in the solutions.

What is the replenishment system of development?

The replenishment system of development requires the addition of a quantity of replenishment solution to the developer to maintain the proper level of solution. When films are removed from the developer solution, they should be removed quickly and the solution on the film drained into the rinse tank. The excess solution should never be allowed to drain back into the developer. It has been estimated that for every forty 14- × 17-inch films 1 gallon of replenisher should be used.

Explain the effect of temperature on the processing cycle.

The rate of development of the radiographic film is dependent upon the temperature of the solution. Therefore, any variation in temperature requires an adjustment in time to maintain a uniform density. It must be noted that at temperatures below 60° F. the action of the hydroquinone almost ceases. When the temperature exceeds 75° F., there is increased activity of the hydroquinone on the film, danger of emulsion softening, and the production of chemical fog.

How often should the developer and fixer in the manual processing cycle be changed?

The developer should be changed when it shows signs of exhaustion or when it no longer develops the exposed silver bromide crystals on the film.

The fixer should be changed when it does not harden the emulsion or when the solution requires more than three minutes to clear the film, the temperature being the same.

How can a film be tested for radiation fog?

The film is developed without exposing it to radiation. Exposure to radiation will cause an increase in density on the film.

What are film abrasions, and how are they caused?

Film abrasions are scratches or similar damage to the film and are caused by careless handling of the film during processing or by dirty rollers in the automatic processor.

Can an underexposed film be corrected by prolonged development?

No. Overdeveloping cannot bring out anything that underexposure failed to put on the film.

With the increase in speed of the automatic processor, the temperature of the solutions had to be increased. What means had to be taken to prevent chemical fog?

To prevent chemical fog from being present at these high temperatures, antifogging agents (aldehydes) had to be added to the developing solution.

To prevent abrasions and softening of the emulsion at high temperatures, what was added to the developing solution?

To prevent abrasion marks on the film and to prevent the emulsion from sticking to the rollers during the processing cycle, solution manufacturers added hardening chemicals to the developing solution.

What are the basic requirements for an efficient, trouble-free automated processing system?

There are three basic components for such a system:

1. A *transport mechanism* will move film sheets through developing, fixing, and washing baths and subsequently through a dryer. Simultaneously, the machine must maintain temperatures and replenish solutions and also provide an adequate air supply properly circulated through the drier.

2. A *system of developing and fixing chemistry* will yield satisfactory sensitometric or radiographic results and also a confluence of their movement through the machine.

3. An *x-ray film* is designed to give good radiographs within the mechanical limitations imposed by the transport system and the required processing chemistry.

The key requirement of such a system, therefore, is compatibility of processor, chemistry, and film. Incompatibility of any one component with the other two will result in marginal performance of the system and cause transport problems or radiographic deficiencies or both.

What aspect of the transport system is considered to be most critical?

The key function of the transport mechanism is to move the sheets of film through all phases of the processing cycle at a uniform rate. Hesitation at any point along the travel path because of the malfunctioning of specific rollers or the main drive system can cause difficulty. If a sheet of film hesitates in the developer for a significant period of time, overdevelopment can occur. This will result in higher-than-normal densities and an increase in fog. In addition, the leading sheet can be overtaken by the following sheet. A jam then becomes imminent. Hesitation in the drying phase wherein the film surfaces pass through a tacky stage is likely to cause the sheet to adhere to a roller and thereby result in a drier jam. It is essential, therefore, that all elements of the drive mechanisms be adequately maintained to ensure uniform travel of the film sheets through all phases of the processing and drying cycles at a constant speed.

In manual processing the role of the processing chemical is to convert a latent radiographic image into a visible image yielding information of diagnostic value. Is this role expanded in automated processing systems?

The chemistry used in automatic processors must do more than control the physical characteristics of the film throughout the entire process, thereby minimizing the possibility of jams, roller wraparounds, roller slippage, and other transport problems. Because of the influence of processing chemicals on both the photographic and physical performance of a sheet of x-ray film, the processing solutions must be constantly maintained at prescribed levels of activity and acidity or alkalinity through carefully controlled replenishment. Over- or under-replenishment caused either by improperly mixed replenishers or by malfunctioning or incorrectly adjusted replenishment systems will adversely affect the physical characteristics of the film and thereby contribute to transport problems. Every periodic maintenance check of the processor should include a careful check of the entire replenishment system.

What film characteristics must be monitored by the film manufacturer to ensure compatibility with automatic processors?

Film manufacturers must exercise a high degree of quality control over both the radiographic (sensitometric) and the physical characteristics of x-ray film. The speed, contrasts, and fog of a film must be within narrow limits before the film can be considered acceptable for use in automated systems. During manufacturing these characteristics are evaluated under the same conditions of time, temperature, and chemical activity that are found in the rapid processing cycles of automatic processors.

In addition, other characteristics known to influence the physical performance of a film are accurately measured. Among those film characteristics of importance in this area are total thickness of the film, thickness uniformity between the front and back emulsion layers, curl, drying rate, swelling characteristics, tackiness, and emulsion hardness.

Basically, therefore, a film must meet two requirements: it must produce high-quality radiographic images, and it must transport satisfactorily through the processor.

The twofold function of the developer in conventional manual processing systems is to swell the gelatinous component of an emulsion, thereby making possible the absorption of chemicals and the subsequent production of a visible image. Has this function been modified in the developers used in automatic processors?

The developers designed for use in automated, high-temperature, short-cycle processors perform essentially the same function as do the conventional developers used in hand processing. In addition, however, machine developers must also restrict emulsion swelling to control the capacity of the emulsion layers to carry the developer over into the next processing bath. This is accomplished by incorporating into the developer a hardening agent that not only limits swelling of the gelatin and thus liquid carryover but also increases the abrasion and resistance of the film surfaces. It also minimizes the scratching and scraping that could occur because of roller-to-film contacts throughout the cycle.

As a consequence of these additional developer requirements, proper replenishment must be ensured at all times. Inadequate developer replenishment can result in excessive swelling and transport difficulties throughout the developing phase of the processing cycle. Furthermore, by not controlling the developer carryover, improper developer replenishment can result in excessive swelling and transport difficulties throughout the developing phase of the processing cycle, and improper developer replenishment can cause an adverse effect on the fixing bath.

What adverse effects can be expected from temperature variations in the developer?

The effects of temperature fluctuations will depend upon the degree of variation from the recommended temperature. Temperatures higher than normal will cause increases in effective film speed, gradient, and fog. Temperatures lower than normal will have an opposite effect. None of these effects is desirable because it will necessitate compensatory modifications in exposure techniques. In addition to these radiographic manifestations of temperature fluctuations, the physical characteristics of the film will change. High temperatures can cause excessive emulsion swelling and a consequent increase in the carryover capacity of the film. This, in turn, will affect the subsequent processing phases.

Standardization of exposure techniques and radiographic quality depends on proper maintenance of recommended temperature of the developer and the other processing baths. Periodic checks on the thermostatic controls of the processor are the best preventative measures that can be taken to minimize "floating" exposure techniques. Proper control of temperature also helps to ensure good transportability of film through the processor.

Can an inadequately replenished fixer affect the image quality of a radiograph?

One function of a fixing solution is to remove all unexposed, undeveloped silver salts from the film. A weak fixing solution cannot accomplish this function in the brief time it takes for a film to be transported through the fixer tank in an automated system. The "finished" radiograph, therefore, contains quantities of undeveloped silver halide crystals having the capability of

printing-out, that is, of being darkened on further exposure to light. This has the effect of reducing radiographic contrast and thereby causing a degradation of image quality. Also the presence of this additional print-out silver creates the esthetically undesirable effect of muddiness.

Does inadequate fixing in any way affect the washing characteristics of an emulsion?

An inadequately fixed film contains quantities of undissolved insoluble silver complexes than cannot be removed from the emulsion in the washing time allotted by the processor design. As a result the washing cycle, which was adequate for a properly fixed film, becomes inadequate for one that was transported through a weak fixing solution or one that was used below the recommended temperature. In such a situation the deficiencies of the system are compounded.

The additive nature of these inadequacies is in itself a basis for carefully monitoring the performance of the replenishment systems.

Can the condition of a fixing bath affect the drying characteristics of a film?

The acidity of the fixer can affect significantly the drying characteristics of a film. At one time during the period between the wet and dry state of a film, the emulsion layers become tacky. While the film is in this condition, the probability is very high that its surfaces will stick to the roller surfaces. The degree of tackiness that occurs is largely dependent upon the pH of the fixer. Films processed through a fixer having a high pH level will become more tacky during drying than will films fixed in a bath at a lower pH. Drier jams can be minimized by controlling the pH of the fixer through maintaining constant, adequate replenishment of that bath.

Does the condition of the fixer affect any characteristics of automatically processed

radiographs other than tackiness during drying?

The archival permanence of radiographs is directly influenced by the condition of the fixing bath. Efficient hypo removal from films during the wash cycle, which is a prerequisite to the archival keeping quality, is dependent to a large measure on the acidity of the fixer. On one hand, films bathed in high pH fixers wash more rapidly and efficiently than those bathed in low pH fixers. On the other hand, high pH fixers tend to produce more tackiness during drying than low pH fixers. Obviously, therefore, a compromise hypo removal must be established and maintained. Consequently it becomes mandatory that the recommended pH level of the fixer be maintained by accurate replenishment if radiographs of archival permanence are to be transported satisfactorily through automatic processors.

In what way can the water supply in a given installation affect a processing system?

The importance of water purity to any photographic processing system becomes evident when consideration is given to the following facts:

1. Usually water from a common source within the x-ray department is used not only to prepare the processing solutions but also to wash the film immediately after fixing. Thus any impurities in the water supply are distributed throughout the entire processing system.
2. The quantity of water used in the system is greater than the chemical constituents of both the developer and the fixer.

Water purity, therefore, should not be considered an insignificant factor, especially in automated, high-speed systems in which it can affect both the photographic and physical performance of a film.

What is water hardness? Can it affect processing in any way?

Hardness is a measure of the calcium and magnesium content of water. Generally water containing more than 100 parts per million of calcium (as calcium carbonate) is considered to be hard.

Hard water usually creates no serious photographic problems. However, it can cause other difficulties. Undesirable precipitates can form in the developer; water spotting and drier streaking can be aggravated; scale can accumulate in the heat exchanger and the tubing within the processor. Scale buildup can affect the efficiency of the replenishment and recirculation systems over a period of time and thereby contribute to transport problems. Therefore, these systems should be carefully checked at frequent intervals at installations located in hardwater areas.

In a given installation the manual processing system requires a fifteen- to thirty-minute wash cycle. The automatic processor in the next room uses the same water supply yet washes the same type of film in about one-tenth that time. How is this possible?

The main function of film washing is the removal of hypo and soluble silver complexes from the emulsion layers. This is accomplished by the diffusing of hypo or by the surrounding water. Such a process can be accelerated by increasing the temperature of the wash bath. This expedient by itself, however, will not accomplish adequate washing because the concentration of hypo in the water quickly comes into balance with that remaining in the film. This stagnant condition must be alleviated by the circulation of large quantities of fresh water through the wash tank, thereby permitting more of the chemicals to diffuse from the emulsion layers.

Automatic processors utilize both of these expedients to reduce washing time to a minimum. They maintain wash water temperatures substantially higher than those used in manual processing systems and require water supplies ranging from 2 to 4 gallons per minute. Less than recommended quantities of wash water will result in insufficient washing and subsequent transport difficulties in the drier.

Periodic maintenance checks should include a flow rate determination of the water supply.

Surface irregularities, visible by reflected light, appear on automatically processed radiographs in varying degrees. What conditions cause these marks?

Areas of varying reflectance characteristics, visible on the surfaces of radiographs, are caused by the drying rate variations. The basic cause for these variations is inherent in the design of roller transport systems. While contacting the film surfaces and thereby moving the sheet through the drier, the drive rollers momentarily prevent the forced air circulating through the chamber from reaching those contact areas. Differential drying and consequently differential surface characteristics result.

Normally these marks are diffuse, inobvious, and do not degrade radiographic quality. Some influencing factors, however, can maximize these marks, thereby making them obvious and esthetically undesirable:

1. Chemical imbalances within the processing system caused by contamination of solutions or erratic replenishment can affect the fixing, washing, and drying characteristics of a film.
2. Drier temperature set at a higher-than-necessary level will aggravate the condition.
3. Hard water can contribute to the problem.
4. Mechanical deficiencies, which cause the film sheets to move erratically rather than uniformly through the drier, will amplify the condition.

Linear bands differing in width but all paralleling the travel path of the film through the processor have become apparent on the surfaces of recent radiographs. Those on the top side of the radiograph vary in number and distribution from those on the bottom side. What is the origin of these bands?

Linear surface drying bands result from the partial obstruction of air flow at given points along the slot of a drier tube. The obstruction is usually an accumulation of dust that effectively blocks one area of the slot and diverts the air flow to either side of the blockage. As the film is transported past this slot, the linear surface area passing the dust accumulation dries at a rate different from that of the adjacent areas. As a result, straight bands of different surface characteristics are produced.

The pattern variation between top and bottom surfaces of a sheet is caused by the fact that each surface is influenced by its respective drier tubes. Therefore a sheet-to-sheet consistency in the top-side pattern as well as a sheet-to-sheet consistency in the bottom-side pattern will be apparent. On the other hand, a top-to-bottom pattern variation will be identifiable. This problem will be eliminated by the clearing of all air tube slots.

What drier temperature is considered optimum?

Drier temperature should be considered to be a controllable variable and not a constant. Essentially, only two drying conditions can be considered constant in well-adjusted automatic processors. These are the quantity of air forced through the drier and the rate of speed at which a sheet of film is transported through that chamber. The quality of the air supply available for use in the drier is not constant. It varies somewhat in temperature and much more so in relative humidity. Likewise the work load imposed upon the drier fluctuates as film sizes vary from 5 × 7 inches to 14 × 17 inches and as film types change from fast films of high silver content to slower films of lower silver content.

In view of these changeable conditions, temperature control becomes a handy tool for regulating the drying capacity of the processor. When the relative humidity of the air supply available for circulation through the drier is high, the drier temperature should be increased to prevent underdrying. On the other hand, the drier temperature should be decreased during the winter months in cold climates to compensate for the low ambient relative humidity and the consequent increase in drying rate.

What are the consequences of underdrying or overdrying a film?

The moisture content of film at a given time affects the hardness and tackiness of the emulsion layers as well as the stiffness, brittleness, and curl characteristics of the sheet as a whole.

Inadequately dried radiographs will exhibit limpness and will be further characterized by relatively soft, swollen emulsion layers, which are tacky to a degree that is dependent upon the state of wetness. Such sheets can jam at the drier exit, stick to a roller during transport through the drier, or stick to each other after exiting into the film receptacle. They are also susceptible to abrasions and scratches.

Overdried radiographs, on the other hand, can exhibit poor brittleness characteristics because of the extreme extraction of moisture from both the emulsion layers and the film base. In addition, the sheets can curl toward one emulsion or the other, depending upon the side-to-side drying differential. This will increase the potential of transport problems.

A film can be considered adequately dried when it exits the drier relatively flat and stiff and exhibits no signs of tackiness or dampness. In adjusting the drier for a given film type and a prevailing set of con-

ditions, the temperature should be lowered progressively until some sign of dampness and limpness appears. The temperature then should be increased progressively until these conditions disappear. The temperature should be maintained at that level or slightly higher for adequate drying.

What characteristics of an x-ray film affect its transportability through a roller-type automatic processor?

Automatic roller-type processors impose the following requirements on x-ray film:

1. Emulsion swelling must be controlled to limit the liquid-carrying capacity of the film. This affects the carryover of solution from one tank to the next and the water load taken into the drier.
2. Emulsion hardness must be kept within prescribed limits to minimize physical damage to the film and to control tackiness during drying.
3. Curl tendencies must be minimized to ensure good tracking of the film from roller to roller, through turnaround and crossover assemblies.

Emulsion swelling and hardness are controlled by both emulsion formulations and processing chemistry. Curl tendencies are controlled by the inherent flatness of the film base and by the careful balancing of the emulsion thicknesses and other characteristics from one side of the sheet to the other.

All film manufacturers monitor each of these influential chemical and physical characteristics of film through careful, quality control programs.

Cleanliness of equipment always has been an important factor in good darkroom procedures. Additional stress has been placed on this aspect of processing since the introduction of automatic processors. In what ways are the automatic systems more critical than the manual systems insofar as cleanliness is concerned?

Great emphasis has been given to equipment cleanliness in the case of automatics for two reasons. First, a lack of cleanliness affects not only the radiographic characteristics of a film but also the transport efficiency of the unit. Secondly, automatic processors have the capacity to affect more sheets of film in a given period of time than do manual systems. Consequently, a large number of radiographs can be rendered unacceptable because of chemical or physical contamination in a short period of time. Thus adequate attention must be given to equipment cleanliness. The clean-up schedules recommended by the processor manufacturer should be followed judiciously.

In manual processing systems physical contaminants such as dust, dirt, lint, and precipitates caused by water impurities usually cause no serious problems. Are automatic processing systems more critical to these impurities?

Physical contaminants can cause several kinds of serious problems in automatic processors. Accumulations of sediments of any kind on transport rollers can affect the tracking of a film through the processor by effectively changing clearance dimensions and, in some cases, contribute to jamming. These accumulations also can be transferred to the films or can produce physical deformations in the film surfaces. In either case the effect is undesirable.

Dust accumulations in the air slots of drier tubes cause nonuniform drying across the film and thereby cause drying marks. Dirt accumulations in the intake or exhaust sections of the drier can alter the capacity of the drier significantly.

The filtering systems of automatic processors, when properly maintained, can be expected to remove physical contaminants from those solutions circulated through them. Accumulations on rollers, however, can be removed only by periodic cleaning. Rollers that cannot be cleaned completely should be replaced.

The investment of time and effort made in properly cleaning and maintaining an automatic processor will return worthwhile dividends in the form of prolonged periods of trouble-free processing.

11 RADIOGRAPHIC QUALITY

What is radiographic quality?

Radiographic quality is a qualitative term that refers to the visibility and sharpness of the images of structural detail. It is controlled or affected by definition, density, contrast, and distortion/magnification.

What is a radiograph?

A radiograph is a permanent photographic record of film of some structure through which some form of ionizing radiation has pased.

What is a diagnostic radiograph?

According to James A. Morgan, a diagnostic radiograph may be defined as the radiograph in which there is sufficient density to show an image of tissue that is adequately penetrated and sharply defined and in which the variations in tissue opacity are sufficiently evident.

What is meant by definition of the anatomic structure?

Definition of the anatomic structure is the sharpness by which the structure has been recorded and by which minimal changes in structure may be detected.

What factors affect radiographic definition?

The following factors affect radiographic definition:

1. The size of the focal spot has much influence on the penumbra effect present in the radiograph. Penumbra is caused by radiation skimming the edges of the object and produces a blurring of the image around its edges. For any given set of circumstances the penumbra effect will vary with the size of the focal spot. In other words, the smaller the focal spot, the less the penumbra or the better the definition.

2. Definition also depends upon the focal-film distance. The sharpest definition is best observed when the focal spot is used at a reasonable target-film distance. When the technologist increases the focal-film distance, the result is almost the same as decreasing the size of the focal spot since the penumbra effect is minimized. Conversely, when the focal-film distance is decreased, the focal spot tends to increase in size.

3. Another factor that contributes to radiographic definition is the object-film distance. To illustrate this point, the technologist can use a light source at any given distance from the object. If the object is flat against a surface, the definition is good. As the object is pulled away from the surface, the outline of the object becomes indistinct. Therefore, it must be concluded that for the best radiographic definition the object should be close to the film.

4. The next factor to be considered is motion. Motion is perhaps the most likely

cause of unsharpness of definition. While it is always too easy to blame the patient for motion on the film, it usually can be traced back to the technologist who failed to give the proper instructions.

Motion may be classified as voluntary or involuntary. Voluntary motion is considered to be the motion that is controlled by the patient under the direction of the technologist. The expression "you moved" seems the easiest to make. It is the technologist who cares who explains the procedure to the patient, explains and demonstrates what needs to be done, and uses any of the immobilizing devices that are necessary to reduce motion. In some instances the necessity for another person to hold the patient may arise. One should always remember that no member of the radiology department should ever hold a person being x-rayed.

Involuntary motion is that which is not stopped by command or immobilizing device. It is associated with the physiologic function of our body, for example heartbeat, peristalsis. It also can be considered as that emanating from very young children. The technologist has no control over this motion except by the means of short exposure time.

5. The final factor of definition can be considered material unsharpness, and it incorporates the film function, the intensifying screen, and the film-screen contact. All medical radiographic film is manufactured to produce the best radiographic detail sharpness. The resolving power of the x-ray is said to be about twenty lines per millimeter.

The intensifying screen may be considered as contributing to the overall lessening of definition. Unsharpness of definition is the result of crystal size and emulsion thickness. The unsharpness of definition has a direct bearing upon the speed of the screens.

Poor screen contact is the result of trapped air between the screens and is not a result of film function. The trapped air between the screens does not permit the screens to come in contact with the film and results in blurring of the image.

What is density?

Density, for the purpose of radiography, may be considered to be the overall blackening of the film. It is the result of a deposit of black metallic silver on the film after exposure and processing. Tissues to be examined are seen as deposits of black metallic silver of various concentrations.

However, a more precise definition of density would be considered as the logarithm of the ratio of light incident to a film to the light transmitted through the film. The formula for such a logarithm is expressed as follows:

$$D = \text{Log}\ \frac{I_o}{I_t}$$

where
D = Density
I_o = Incident light to the film
I_t = Transmitted light through the film

A densitometer will provide an accurate measurement of light through the film.

What is proper density considered to be?

Proper density is considered to be that amount of black metallic silver properly distributed over the film to make visible the structural details of the anatomic image. From this statement it can then be inferred that the absence of black metallic silver or the greater deposit of silver will tend to obliterate the tissue details of the image.

How do you expain the difference of densities on the film?

Whereas density is considered to be the overall blackening on the film, we must also realize that it is the amount of radiation absorbed by the film. As the radiation beam passes through the body, parts of the beam are absorbed by various anatomic tissues. The absorption by these tissues reduces the total radiation beam that reaches the film. The resultant radiation produces several different deposits of silver upon the film. Each deposit will be different, depending upon the strength of the radiation beam. The greater the deposit of silver, the less light will come through when viewed upon an illuminator.

How is density controlled?

1. Density is controlled primarily by milliampere-seconds, or mas. Milliampere-seconds is the product of milliamperage multiplied by the time in seconds. A direct relationship exists between the amount of density and the change in milliampere-seconds. When the amount of energy to the film is doubled, the result is a doubling of the density upon the film. However, in viewing the finished radiograph the technologist must determine whether the density or the penetration is adequate. No amount of density change will compensate for the lack of penetration of the part. To establish correct density settings for any technique there first must be correct penetration. The use of milliampere-seconds is a quantitative factor in the production of density.

2. Density also is controlled in part by kilovoltage, or kvp. As higher energy is applied to the x-ray tube, the resultant radiation output is of shorter and more penetrating wavelength. The more penetrating the wavelength, the greater the amount of primary radiation reaching the film will be because of less part absorption. Thus the increased kilovoltage produces a greater density upon the film. Whereas it was noted that the effect of milliampere-seconds upon the density was proportional, it must be stated that the effect of kilovoltage is not the same. At this point the technologist should be made aware of the rule of thumb, which states that an increase of ten in kilovoltage will cause a reduction of one half in the milliampere-sec-

onds. However, this rule is only permissible with exposures above 60 kilovolts.

3. Distance also affects density. If the light source of a flashlight is pointed close to the object, the light density at that place is bright. As the light source is withdrawn, the area loses its brightness, and the rays are spread over a larger area, thus reducing the energy and light. X-rays are similar to this illustration. As the distance from the film is increased, the width of the beam increases, and more area is radiated with the same amount of primary radiation. This means that a larger surface is being exposed with no increase in radiation. Therefore, the result is less radiation for each given area of the larger film. The total amount of radiation is the same, but each square inch receives less radiation than a comparable square inch of a smaller film.

What is radiographic contrast?

Radiographic contrast is the difference in densities that makes the anatomic images and related structures visible. A good radiograph is one in which there is good distribution of black metallic silver over the contrast scale. The contrast scale is determined by the number of different densities that are seen on the film from the white to the black. Contrast cannot occur unless two or more densities exist on the film.

Are other types of contrast to be considered in the overall radiographic picture?

Yes. Other types of contrast that affect radiographic contrast are developer contrast, tissue or subject contrast, and film contrast.

1. The most common developer in use today is the sodium carbonate developer, which produces a long-scale contrast when used under proper conditions. However, a developer using sodium hydroxide produces an image of greater contrast than that produced by sodium carbonate. The type of contrast is inherent in the manu-

factured solution. The technologist must also realize that a change in contrast can occur with a change in the time of development and in the temperature.

2. Tissue or subject contrast is signified by the difference in the intensity of the radiation emerging from that particular anatomic region. The difference in density levels depends upon the absorption of radiation by the part and that radiation reaching the film. Radiation having the characteristic of a long wavelength has little penetrating power and produces few densities because of tissue absorption, while radiation of short wavelength produces many densities because of its penetration power.

3. Film contrast is that which has been manufactured with inherent contrast characteristics. Film contrast is actually a graph of density measured against the logarithm of a known exposure. With the two types of film in use, screen film is more sensitive to the blue-violet light of the intensifying screens and less sensitive to the action of direct exposure. The film characteristic is thus that it presents a higher contrast where exposed to the intensifying screen. The direct exposure or nonscreen film is especially sensitive to the action of direct x-ray exposure. The film is manufactured with a thicker emulsion and provides a higher contrast than screen film. It should never be used with screens.

What factors control contrast?

The primary factor controlling radiographic contrast is kilovoltage, or kvp. We are led to believe that the scale of densities determines the radiographic contrast. These densities are the result of the absorption of radiation by anatomic parts. The absorption or nonabsorption of radiation is determined by the intensity of radiation or wavelength. The wavelength is determined by the utilization of kilovoltage. When kilovoltages of low energy are used, the radiation is of long wavelength and may be easily absorbed by tissue. Thus, only a

small degree of remnant radiation may reach the film and become absorbed. The difference in tonal densities are great, and only a few densities are present. This represents short-scale contrast. On the other hand, when high energy kilovoltage is employed, the radiation produced is in the form of short wavelengths and penetrates more easily. The remnant radiation is more easily recorded as a difference in density upon the film. The difference between the densities is small, yet distinct, and produces a radiograph of long-scale contrast.

Milliampere-seconds in conjunction with kilovoltage have an effect upon contrast. With low kilovoltage and high milliamperage-seconds, a film of high contrast is produced, whereas, conversely, low contrast is produced with low milliamperage-seconds and high kilovoltage. Therefore, it must be noted that any increase or decrease in kilovoltage may result in a change in the milliamperage-second factor to compensate for the effect upon density.

A factor not to be overlooked in the control of contrast is fog. Fog is considered to be an extra layer of density superimposed upon the original density. It adds an objectionable density since it inhibits the visibility of the radiographic image and destroys the ability to differentiate the various densities on the film.

Name some kinds of fog and their prevention.

Fog may take a variety of forms and affects contrast. Age, chemical, light, heat, and safelight fog are just a few to be mentioned.

Age fog may be prevented by using the films with the oldest expiration date stamped on the film package first. Films should be stored so that packages with the oldest expiration dates are in the front.

Chemical fog is caused by developer chemicals and should be controlled by proper time and temperature. Also, contamination and oxidation of the chemicals should be checked.

Light fog may be controlled and prevented by making sure that all darkrooms and loading rooms are not subject to white light leaks. Films should never be opened in the white light, and film bin drawers should be securely shut.

Heat fog is prevented by not placing films either in cassettes or storage close to heating pipes. Films should be stored in a cool, dry place.

Safelight fog is prevented by using the correct wattage bulb and not allowing the exposed film to be subjected to the safelight for long periods of time before processing.

What is secondary radiation fog?

Secondary radiation fog is radiation that is given off by the parts of the body being radiographed and is characteristic of the part being struck. The secondary radiation strikes the film and produces a uniform density on the film.

Secondary radiation fog is produced by the primary radiation utilized and is partially controlled by kilovoltage. Also it is produced by the various tissues of the patients. Tissues that contain a high percentage of fluid tend to produce more scattered radiation than those that have little fluid.

How can secondary radiation fog be controlled or reduced?

Secondary radiation fog may be controlled or reduced by using only the amount of kilovoltage that will adequately penetrate the area thickness and by restricting the size of the area irradiated, using the smallest beam restrictor possible. The use of a grid is probably the most effective type of control. The higher the grid ratio and the greater the number of lead strips per inch, the more effective the grid will be.

The addition of filtration into the path of the beam to absorb or attenuate the longer

wavelengths will contribute to the reduction of secondary radiation and subsequently the fog level.

Under what conditions may secondary radiation fog be produced on a film?

Secondary radiation fog may be produced on a film when the part is close to the film. The part that is close to the film will not allow the production of fog within the image but may produce fog surrounding it.

If the object to be radiographed is placed at a distance from the film, the secondary radiation is allowed to penetrate to the film.

What is distortion of the radiographic image?

Distortion, as we view it, is the perversion of the true shape of an image when radiographed. It usually becomes either elongated or foreshortened. The distortion of the image places the relationship of one part of the body in unnatural form and shape. The technologist must remember that all the body parts are not completely round or flat and that because of this configuration there will always be some phase of distortion. The distortion of the anatomic part is controlled by correct object-tube alignment.

What is magnification of the radiographic image?

Magnification of the radiographic image is defined as the enlargement, or increase in size, of the image on the radiograph. It must be understood that all magnification is not bad and objectionable. Of necessity there will always be some magnification, but, if there is distinction of good radiographic definition, it will be tolerated. The degree of enlargement of the radiographed objective will be dependent upon the focal-film distance and the object-film distance.

What are the four basic factors of exposure controlled by the technologist?

The four basic factors of exposure are kilovoltage, milliamperage, time, and distance.

What is meant by magnification factor?

Magnification factor may be defined as the ratio of the object width to the image width and is formularized as follows:

$$\text{Magnification factor} = \frac{\text{Image width}}{\text{Object width}}$$

What is meant by the percentage of magnification?

The percentage of magnification is the percentage of enlargement of the radiographic image as measured with the original object. It can be set in the formula that follows:

$$\text{Percentage of magnification} = \frac{\text{Image width} - \text{Object width} \times 100}{\text{Object width}}$$

What is meant by the "heel" effect? What is its use?

The intensity of radiation from a target differs according to the various angles of emission. Thus the heel effect is a variation of intensity of radiation along the longitudinal axis of the tube. The intensity of radiation tends to fade out rapidly from the area of the central ray toward the anode side of the tube. The intensity of radiation continues to expand and slowly diminishes from the area of the central ray toward the cathode side of the tube.

It is justifiably used in areas where there is a need to balance densities caused by differences in tissue, for example, the upper thoracic area.

What radiographic factors are considered to be quantitative and qualitative?

The milliamperage determines the number of electrons crossing from the cathode to the anode in any given length of time. Milliamperage denotes the exposure rate and thus is quantitative.

The kilovoltage is the electric potential applied to the cathode to drive the free electrons to the anode. The degree of potentiality determines the wavelength form of the x-ray beam. Low potential produces a beam of long wavelength, while higher potential produces short wavelengths. Since the form of the wavelength controls the penetration of the beam, kilovoltage is said to be qualitative.

What is the latent image?

The latent image may be described as the image that is invisible to the eye that has been created on the radiographic film through the medium of light or x-rays. The latent image becomes visible when processed. When struck by radiation, the silver bromide crystals become positively charged silver ions and negatively charged bromine ions. The emulsion, when it is manufactured, is chemically treated to cause sensitization specks to be produced on some crystals. These sensitization specks can only be affected by radiation exposure or light. With the radiographic exposure, electrons of the bromine are set free and become attached to the neutral speck, transforming it into a negative charge. This negative charge attracts a silver ion and becomes neutral again. This process continues during the length of exposure. When enough silver has been attracted to the speck, it acts as a development area and a latent image is formed.

What is screen unsharpness?

When radiation is applied to a cassette bearing intensifying screens, the energy is converted into fluorescent light. The image lines produced by the excitation of the crystals produce lines that are broader than the lines produced by direct radiation, and the image light of the crystals reacts upon one another in enhancing or detracting from the sharpness. Because of this diffusion of image light, intensifying screens produce loss of image sharpness.

What does the term "umbra" denote in radiography?

In radiography umbra is considered to be the image radiographed with clearly marked margins of extremity.

What does the term "penumbra" denote?

Penumbra is used to denote the hazy, ill-defined edge of the object radiographed and can be used to measure radiographic unsharpness.

What is a step wedge and for what is it used?

A step wedge is a homogenous object of aluminum made in the formation of a series of steps, usually from one to ten, with each succeeding higher step increased by one thickness over the lower one. In this manner, if the first step contains one thickness of aluminum, the last will contain ten thicknesses. The step wedge is used to test the efficiency of the machine and to control density.

What factors other than contrast, detail, and magnification/distortion directly affect density?

The following factors directly affect density and only indirectly affect contrast.
1. Thickness of part
2. Opacity of tissue
3. Pathology
4. Compression
5. Respiration
6. Focal-film distance

What factors directly affect contrast?

The factors that directly affect contrast and indirectly affect density are:
1. Bucky
2. Cones
3. Screens
4. Cardboard holders

5. Filters
6. Film

Are there factors present that may affect both density and contrast?

Yes. Processing of the film and the radiographic efficiency of the equipment used are two factors that will affect both density and contrast.

What is the inverse square law, and how is it expressed in formula?

The inverse square law states that the intensity of radiation varies inversely with the square of the distance and may be expressed in the formula that follows:

$$I_1 : I_2 :: D_2^2 : D_1^2$$

Is there a relationship between the exposure time and the distance for radiographic exposures?

The exposure time required for any given radiographic exposure is directly proportional to the square of the focal-film distance and may be expressed as follows:

$$T1 : T2 :: D1^2 : D2^2$$

Explain the relationship between the milliamperage and the time in radiography.

The milliamperage required for any given radiographic exposure is inversely proportional to the time of that exposure. It may be expressed as the following:

$$MA_1 : MA_2 :: T_2 : T_1$$

What is a cone?

In radiographic work a cone is a metal, cone-shaped tube having a small aperture at one end and a particular diameter opening at the other end. The cone is placed in the beam of x-ray close to the tube opening to restrict the area of x-ray radiation.

What are the uses of diaphragms in radiography?

The diaphragm is a beam-restricting device and is constructed of a sheet of lead or steel out of which a hole has been cut to permit radiation to pass.

What are collimators?

Collimators are beam-restricting devices constructed of variable apertures. They are usually made of double diaphragm construction (one on top of the other), with each one capable of delineating the outline of the beam restriction. Most collimators are now equipped with some beam-centering device for further accuracy by the technologist.

Of what use is the cone, the diaphragm, and the collimator?

These are used to confine the beam to the immediate area under examination and thus minimize the secondary radiation within the patient's body by limiting the volume of tissue exposed. The result is greatly increased contrast, which makes radiographic detail more plainly visible.

Does the diameter of a cone control the degree of efficiency or effectiveness?

No. The determining factor is the area of the field of radiation, and this depends on the diameter of the cone, the length of the cone, and the focal-film distance.

Is there an advantage in using a cone with a Potter-Bucky diaphragm?

The use of a cone may be definitely advantageous. No Potter-Bucky diaphragm is 100% effective in absorbing secondary radiation. The cone, by limiting the size of the field being irradiated, decreases the amount of secondary radiation that may be set up. For instance, in radiography of the gallbladder, a decided difference can be demonstrated between radiographs taken with a cone and without a cone employing a Potter-Bucky diaphragm.

Explain the construction of a cassette.

A casette is a framelike film container used as a mounting for intensifying screens. The front is constructed of a low x-ray absorption material and faces the x-ray tube during exposure. The cassette's metal back is hinged for easy opening and closing. Felt padding and a thin layer of lead foil are placed between the back screen and metal back to prevent light leakage and to assure the absorption of back scatter radiation. Locks are placed on the metallic back to hold the casette closed and assure proper contrast between the screens and x-ray film.

Explain the construction of a cardboard holder.

The cardboard holder is constructed of two pieces of specially constructed cardboard or plastic to form a light-tight envelope. The cardboards are joined together at the top and have a special envelope that is made for the insertion of the film attached to the back portion. Between the envelope and the back portion is often found a small piece of thin lead foil to prevent back scatter from reaching the film. A locking device for joining the two open ends completes the construction.

What are intensifying screens?

Intensifying screens are radiolucent cardboard or plastic coated screens with a layer of chemical material suspended in a suitable emulsion that will fluoresce when penetrated by radiation. One side of the cardboard or plastic is covered by a high reflectant surface to which the phosphor layer is coated. The entire screen is covered with a thin coating of protective material, and the edges are sealed to protect them from moisture.

Describe the phosphor layer of the intensifying screen.

The phosphor coat of an intensifying screen is composed of many layers of fluorescent crystals. These crystals must be thoroughly dispersed prior to application by many hours of mixing in a solution consisting of solvents and a clear binder. This mixture is then coated at a predetermined thickness on a suitable support. As the solvent evaporates the coat becomes firm and eventually hard.

The speed of the screen is determined by the type of phosphor used, thickness of the active layers, size of phosphors, and ability of the backing to reflect light. Screens having thicker emulsion are faster, within limits, because there are more crystals to emit light It is, however, axiomatic that the thicker the phosphor layer, the poorer the detail.

Describe the screen backing necessary for use in intensifying screens.

The screen backing usually consists of a high-quality cord stock of uniform thickness made either from wood pulp or cotton cuttings. Certain plastic materials have also been used, but care must be utilized to prevent static discharges. The stock must be free from inclusions of metal, fiber, or other radiopaque foreign substances. It also must possess great dimensional stability and adequate firmness to lend the desired support. The quality must be such that no discoloration will occur during the life of the screen; otherwise the screen may lose speed. The surface adjacent to the phosphor layer is coated with a highly reflecting compound such as titanium dioxide to enhance the overall speed of the screen. The back surface is usually provided with a moisture-proof seal coat to inhibit moisture penetration.

Explain the purpose of the protective coating on the intensifying screen.

This coating is very important since, barring accident, the service of the screen depends on it. Its purpose is to protect the phosphor layer. It must not be too thick because the film should be as near as possible to the source of light. This fact is readily apparent since the nearer the film is to the crystals, the better the definition. The protective coat should not be too thin, or the useful life of the screen will be short. Also this coat should be hard enough to prevent foreign material from being imbedded in its surface. If it is not, artifacts on the film may be the direct penalty. The surface should be moisture-proof, resistant to abrasions and stains, and readily cleanable. Resistance to abrasions is particularly important because screens are subject to considerable wear as cassettes are loaded and unloaded and as pressure is applied in closing the cassettes.

Why is the edge seal necessary in manufacturing screens?

The purpose of this seal is to join the front protective surface and the back moisture-proof coat, thus preventing the penetration of moisture through the edges. Without this seal and without suitable front and back coats, the screen may become wrinkled because of absorption of moisture. Sealing also helps to prevent chipping of the phosphor layer, particularly at the corners.

Are there different types of intensifying screens?

Yes. Presently three types of intensifying screens, based primarily upon their application and speed, are mainly used. They are classified as high-speed, medium-speed, and slow-speed.

With the need to reduce exposure to the patient yet continue to exhibit proper radiographic detail consistent with proper diagnosis, interest has been demonstrated in the use of high-speed screens. These high-speed screens utilizing large size crystals are manufactured under various trade names, such as Superspeed, H. V., Ultra speed, and Radelin TF. Speed may vary widely from one manufactured screen to another. The better screens have a relative exposure factor of 0.5 as compared to medium-speed screens, depending upon the kilovolts peak employed and the absorption of the object being radiographed.

The medium-speed screens are generally used in radiographic procedures. They are between the high-speed and slow-speed screens. They are manufactured under various trade names, such as Universal, Mid-speed, General Purpose, Par-Speed, and Radelin T. It has been established through wide usage that medium screens possess the best balance between speed and detail for most radiographic purposes. The medium-speed screen is frequently used as a standard and assigned an exposure factor of 1.

The slower speed screens render significantly better detail than medium- or high-speed screens. These screens have the smallest sized crystals. They are manufactured under the following names: Fine grain, High definition, Detail, High Resolution, and Ultra Detail. The exposure factors necessary to obtain a specific result may vary as much as two to four times between the various makes of screens. The use of these screens are indicated in bone radiography, in magnification techniques, and in other instances in which maximum detail is desired.

What are fluoroscopic screens?

Fluoroscopic screens are special viewing screens made from zinc cadmium sulfide. This phosphor fluoresces within the maximum sensitivity range of the well-adapted eye. Fluoroscopic examinations permit the observation of anatomic parts at rest or in motion.

What is the difference between the fluoroscopic screen and the intensifying screen?

The main difference between these two screens is primarily in the use of chemical phosphors. The intensifying screen uses the chemical phosphor, calcium tungstate,

which fluoresces with a blue-violet light when exposed to x-ray. The fluoroscopic screen utilizes the phosphor zinc cadmium sulfide, which fluoresces with a yellow-green light when exposed to x-rays.

What is a phosphor?

Phosphors are luminescent or fluorescent chemicals that derive their name from the Greek word meaning "light bearer." They are crystalline in nature. They have the ability of absorbing energy in one form and converting it to another, that is, of absorbing and converting x-rays to visible light. Therefore, phosphors are converters of energy, and this conversion is called luminescence or fluorescence.

Is there a difference between fluorescence and phosphorescence?

Fluorescence, or luminescence, is the emission of visible light by a crystal when subjected to an activating source. Phosphorescence is the emission of light by a crystal after the activating source has ceased.

What does the term "afterglow," or "screen lag," mean?

This is a condition in which the screen continues to emit light after the x-ray source has ceased to be active.

Why is calcium tungstate used in intensifying screens?

Calcium tungstate crystals are used in intensifying screens for the following reasons:
1. The spectral emission is in the blue and ultraviolet spectrum.
2. It has excellent response in the kilovoltage range employed in medical radiography.
3. It is stable in that its characteristics neither change when subjected to the type of x-ray exposure used in radiography nor change with the passage of time.

4. Uniform quality can be produced under proper manufacturing conditions to meet rigid requirements of crystal size, efficiency, and freedom from afterglow.

What were the disadvantages of the first manufactured screens?

The disadvantages of the first manufactured screens were as follows:
1. Graininess, caused by the use of large crystals
2. Objectionable afterglow, or screen lag, because of the impurities in the chemicals
3. Lack of crystal uniformity and manufacturing uniformity
4. The absence of a protective coating that was cleanable

What is a photofluorographic screen?

The photofluorographic, or photoradiographic, screen is a screen coated with either zinc sulfide or zinc cadmium sulfide crystals and placed within a lightproof hood, which also houses a camera lens. The screen is used in mass radiography, and, when the x-ray exposure is made, the screen lights up with the patient's image. Through the means of the camera lens the image is recorded on a smaller film (70 mm. or 4 × 5 inches cut film). Therefore, the resulting image is a photograph of the fluoroscopic image. The zinc sulfide screen is used with blue-sensitive film, and the zinc cadmium sulfide screen is used with green-sensitive film.

What effect will dirt on the intensifying screen have on the finished radiograph?

Dust, dirt particles, and stains, if allowed to collect on the surfaces of the screen, will cause extraneous shadows to be visualized on the radiographic image.

How can the degree of intensification produced by a screen be determined?

With all other factors remaining constant, compare the exposure time required to produce a density of 1.0 on a given part, taken with a regular film in a cardboard holder, to that of a regular film with intensifying screens.

How is speed determined in an intensifying screen?

The speed of the screen is determined by the size of the fluorescent crystal and the thickness of the phosphor layer. In general, fast screens use larger crystals than do those in slower screens. Fig. 7 shows the relative size of the crystals and illustrates their "spread of light" during x-ray excitation to adjacent areas including the film emulsion.

Describe the care needed for a fluoroscopic screen.

Since fluoroscopic screens are not subject to wear and tear, their useful life is long. However, certain precautions must be taken to ensure maximum life and effectiveness. The phosphors used in such screens may discolor if subjected to more than moderate exposure to ultraviolet light, either from sunlight or artificial sources. It is recommended that the screen be protected by a dark cloth when not in use.

Fluoroscopic screens are mounted under lead glass with dustproof tape. Since the tape is not moistureproof, care should be exercised to prevent moisture from coming into contact with the screen. If liquid is spilled on the screen, it should be wiped off immediately to prevent staining and possible warping of the screen. Periodic cleaning of the lead glass to remove finger marks and dust is recommended.

Describe the care needed for an intensifying screen.

Satisfactory performance and useful life of any intensifying screen is dependent upon proper handling, periodic inspection, and cleaning. When a cassette is used, it accumulates bits of film, felt, lint, and dust,

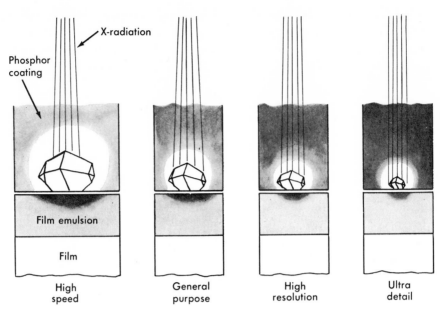

Fig. 7. Effect of crystal size on detail. (Courtesy U.S. Radium Corporation, Radelin Division.)

which are deposited as air is sucked in and forced out in the loading process. It is suggested that a regular inspection schedule be maintained.

Cleaning frequency depends upon usage and concentration of dust in the atmosphere.

What is the effect of temperature upon the intensifying screen?

We may all agree that with temperature changes chemical activity usually changes. As the developer temperature rises, we expect a more rapid excitation of the exposed film. However, this is not true when dealing with the luminescence of the calcium tungstate phosphor. As the temperature rises, the efficiency of the screen decreases.

Within the temperature limits of the temperate zone, these opposing phenomena counterbalance each other and no change in radiographic technique need be made.

Where extremes of temperature are encountered, correction of x-ray factors is required. In hot climates where the temperature may reach 110° F., the basic mas must be increased by approximately 20% to maintain density.

At temperatures below normal 14° F., the opposite is true. Under these conditions the basic mas must be decreased by 25 to 30 percent to maintain proper density.

Do intensifying screens have the same characteristics at all kvp values?

Intensifying screens do not have the same characteristics at all kvp values. The speed, or intensifying factor, is dependent upon the character of the radiation reaching it and upon the characteristics of the chemicals comprising it. In those screens that are used for radiographic work, the intensifying factor at lower kilovoltages is less than that at the higher kilovoltages. The intensification properties of screens increase as the kvp is increased, although not in direct proportion.

What is meant by poor screen contact?

Screens should be in good contact with the film over its entire surface. Failure to adhere to this condition results in poor screen contact. Some causes of poor film-screen contact are as follows:

1. Warping of the cassette front
2. Wrinkled screen caused by penetration of moisture
3. Foreign bodies under the screen, causing uneven pressure
4. Cracked cassette frame or broken hinge
5. Trapped moist air in cassette in extremely humid areas

How do you test for poor screen contact?

Poor screen contact may be checked by radiographing a fine wire mesh, ⅛ to ¼ inch brass or copper, which has the same dimensions as the cassette. If there is good film-screen contact, the image of the wire mesh will be sharp. When the film-screen contact is poor, the image will be fuzzy.

What is meant by screen grain?

Screen grain is usually caused by the presence of oversize crystals of calcium tungstate in the intensifying screen. It is recognized by small, irregular spots having the appearance of freckles on the x-ray film.

How would a technologist determine whether an artifact on the finished radiograph was a result of a defect on the screen or foreign to the patient?

Since a defect on either the screen or the patient would most likely produce an area of light density on the radiograph, another radiograph using a different cassette should be taken. Absence of the lightened area on the second film would eliminate the possibility of its being attributed to the patient. Therefore, the screens should be inspected for the defect.

Are there disadvantages to using intensifying screens?

With the increase of the object-film distance when using the screen in the Bucky, radiographic detail is lost. With the use of high-speed screens and large crystal, radiographic detail is lost. However, the gain in the short exposure time is compensation for the loss in definition.

Draw a cross section of an intensifying screen.

See Fig. 8.

What is a Potter-Bucky diaphragm?

In 1913 Guston Bucky invented the grid diaphragm but was not successful because this grid had to be used in the stationary position. Dr. Hollis Potter made the grid applicable to radiographic procedures by placing it in motion during the rate of exposure. This motion caused the grid lines to be blurred out of the image. Thus the grid and mechanism under the tabletop now is known as the Potter-Bucky diaphragm.

What is the purpose of the Bucky grid?

The Bucky grid was designed to filter out undesirable secondary radiation, which hinders the visibility of good radiographic detail.

What is a grid?

A grid is a device used for filtering the unwanted secondary radiation and is constructed of alternate strips of lead and x-ray translucent material. It is placed between the patient and the film. The radiolucent material should provide stability and yet have a minimum of absorption of the useful primary radiation.

What are the various types of grids?

Grids are classified as parallel, focused, or cross-hatch.

In a parallel grid all of the lead strips are placed parallel to each other and perpendicular to the face of the grid. Thus any line projected from the edge of the lead strip would not meet at any point

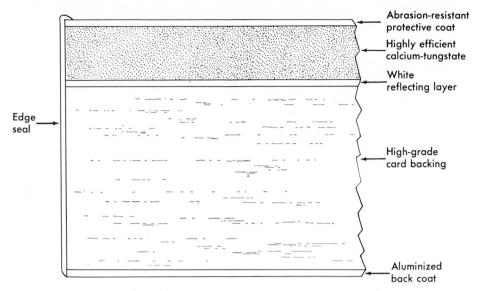

Abrasion-resistant
protective coat

Highly efficient
calcium-tungstate

White
reflecting layer

Edge
seal

High-grade
card backing

Aluminized
back coat

Fig. 8. Cross section of Radelin intensifying screen. (Courtesy U.S. Radium Corporation, Radelin Division.)

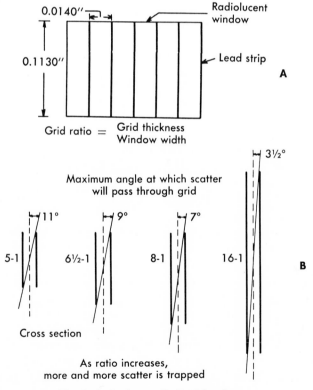

Radiolucent
window

0.0140″

0.1130″

Lead strip

A

Grid ratio = $\dfrac{\text{Grid thickness}}{\text{Window width}}$

Maximum angle at which scatter
will pass through grid

11°   9°   7°   3½°

5-1   6½-1   8-1   16-1

B

Cross section

As ratio increases,
more and more scatter is trapped

Fig. 9. A, Grid ratio. **B,** Grid details.

at any distance from the grid. The parallel grid permits long focal-film distances to be used but contributes to grid cutoff at the shorter distances.

The focused grid is comprised of lead strips angled so that lines drawn from the edge of the lead strips converge at a definite point and distance from the grid. The lead strips in the center of the grid are perpendicular, but as they progress toward the lateral edge from each side of center the lead strips are angled progressively more and more.

The cross-hatch grid is composed of two conventional grids superimposed upon each other; the lead strips of one are at right angles to the lead strips of the other. Thus it is said that a cross-hatch grid of 5:1 ratio has the effective cleanup of a 10:1 ratio grid.

Are there disadvantages or limitations to using the cross-hatch grid?

The cross-hatch grid, because of its design, has excellent cleanup but does have limitations or disadvantages in use. Because the lead strips are at right angles to each other, the tube centering must be accurate to avoid grid cutoff at the edges. Because of the grid construction, the tube cannot be angled more than a few degrees from the perpendicular. A complete cutoff of radiation reaching the film may result if the tube is angled more than 5 degrees from the perpendicular or horizontal direction of the x-ray beam.

What is grid radius?

Grid radius is defined as that distance from the lead strips of the grid to the point (x-ray source) when all the lines will converge. The distance should be measured perpendicularly from this point to the surface of the grid. All focused grids have a specific grid radius to be used for minimal interference of radiation reaching the film.

What is grid ratio?

Grid ratio may be defined as the ratio of the height of the lead strips to the width of the radiolucent spacers between the strips. The higher the grid ratio, the greater the proportionate height of the lead strips will be as compared to the width of the interspaces. In an 8:1 ratio grid the lead strip is eight times higher than the width of the space between it.

What effect does the grid ratio have on the radiograph?

As the grid ratio increases, more and more secondary radiation is trapped by the lead strips; fog is reduced, and radiographic contrast is increased.

Compare the effects of grid ratio on absorption of radiation, density, and contrast.

The x-ray absorption of high-ratio grids will be greater than that of low-ratio grids. The difference between the two can be compensated by the increase of exposure factors for the high-ratio grid.

From the standpoint of density, the grid of higher ratio will absorb a greater percentage of radiation, both primary and secondary. The films taken with it will be lighter than those taken with a low-ratio grid.

Considering contrast, the high-ratio grid eliminates a higher percentage of secondary radiation and will produce films with greater contrast.

A radiograph is exposed and processed, and, when viewed, a lesser density appears on one side when compared to the other side. Explain its cause.

The difference in densities from one side of the film to the other may have been caused by the following:

1. The radiographic tube may have been off-center in relation to the center of the table.
2. The radiographic tube may have

been angled crosswise in relation to the lead strips.

3. The Bucky may not have been level in the table, or the table itself may not have been level.

What is the importance of lines per inch in grid construction?

The number of lead strips per inch has an important bearing on the efficiency of the grid. Lines per inch simply means the number of lead strips per inch across the grid. The more strips per inch, the thinner the lead strips will be. As the grid ratio is maintained, the lines per inch increase the danger of having the lead strips become so thin that their absorption quality will be lacking and higher energy radiation will not be stopped.

How are grid lines caused on a radiograph?

The appearance of grid lines on a radiograph are objectionable. The following are several causes of these grid lines:

1. Grid lines may be caused by having the exposure start before the grid has reached full travel speed.
2. They may be caused by the continuance of the exposure after the grid has slowed down or stopped.
3. Grid lines appear when there is uneven movement of the grid, such as jerky motion.
4. Lines may be caused when the tube is not centered to the center of the grid.
5. The lines appear when the proper grid radius is either decreased or increased beyond the proper operating distance.

Why is the focal-film distance such an important factor in the use of the focused grid?

When the focal spot of the tube is placed at the proper radial distance from the grid, the width of the space between the lead strips is open fully in relation to the x-ray beam. Since these spaces are of equal width, the greatest amount of energy will reach the film, and there will be an equal distribution of the energy.

What is meant by grid specification?

Grid specifications are considered to be those data recommended by the International Commission on Radiologic Units in Handbook 89 to specify the characteristics of focused grids.

1. Number of lines per inch
2. Focal-film distance of the grid
3. Limits of the grid focal-film distance
4. Contrast improvement factor of the grid

However, only the first three specifications are included on the label of the grid.

What is the contrast improvement factor in the grid?

It has already been stated that the efficiency of the grid improves the radiographic contrast. The contrast improvement factor may be defined as the relationship of the contrast with a grid divided by the contrast without the grid. It may be expressed in a formula as follows:

$$CIF = \frac{\text{X-ray contrast with a grid}}{\text{X-ray contrast without a grid}}$$

However, with all factors being equal, the contrast improvement factor will vary as the kvp, field size, and anatomic thickness of part change.

In converting a nongrid technique to a grid technique, we must either increase the mas or the kvp because of the absorption of the grid. Can you give the approximate conversion factor for the various grid ratios utilizing mas as the conversion factor?

From nongrid to	5:1 use 2 times mas
	6:1 use 3 times mas
	8:1 use 4 times mas
	10:1 use 5 times mas
	12:1 use 5 times mas
	16:1 use 6 times mas

In converting nongrid techniques utilizing kvp as the conversion factor, what would be the approximate conversions?

From nongrid to 5:1 add 8 kvp
6:1 add 12 kvp
8:1 add 20 kvp
12:1 add 23 kvp
16:1 add 25 kvp

What is a filter?

A filter may be defined as any material that, when placed in the path of the primary radiation, will absorb a part of that radiation. The filters generally used in medical radiography are made of aluminum or copper. They are placed in the filter slot of the x-ray tube just below the exit portal of the tube. Every x-ray tube has filtration built into it. This is called inherent filtration. The inherent filtration consists of the glass envelope of the tube insert, the oil surrounding the insert, and the glass exit portal. It is equivalent to 0.5 mm. of aluminum at tubes rated for use of up to 100 kvp and to 1 mm. of aluminum at tubes rated for use above 100 kvp. The National Committee on Radiation Protection and Measurements recommends the addition of 2 mm. more of aluminum filtration to the tubes.

What is a compensating filter?

A compensating filter is a device constructed and used in medical radiography so that anatomic parts of various thicknesses may be made more properly visible on the finished radiograph. Such filters are made of aluminum, copper, or barium plastic. The principle of the filter is to make possible the selection of an exposure that will give penetration to the heavier part yet, through absorption by the filter, will give satisfactory exposure to the thin part, thus allowing a uniform density to be present over the entire area of the radiograph.

Can you explain the mechanics of the Potter-Bucky diaphragm?

It is well understood that the Bucky moves during the exposure to prevent grid lines from appearing on the film. In the single-stroke type of grid the Bucky is cocked by the technologist; that is, the Bucky is pulled to one side of the table by a lever and thus puts a spring under tension. When the grid is released, the spring pulls the grid across the table. The motion of the grid is controlled by a piston acting either against oil in a cylinder or compressed air in a chamber. The rate of travel is controlled by the passage of oil into a second chamber through a predetermined channel size or by the escape of air through a predetermined hole. The timing device is set by the technologist.

The grid travels about 2 inches across the table and usually reaches its maximum speed after traveling about ⅕ inch. It is at this instant that the exposure should start. The exposure should terminate before the grid stops moving at the steady speed and before reaching the full travel of 2 inches.

What is the reciprocating Bucky?

The reciprocating Bucky is a grid operated by a motor-driven mechanism. It continually oscillates back and forth across the table without any manual cocking. Each stroke of the grid requires about 1¼ seconds in time. The grid movement is initiated before the exposure starts and continues to operate as long as the motor drive is activated.

It has been said that radiographs exposed through a moving grid should show no evidence of grid lines when the grid is properly used. From this statement of fact what radiographic premises can be assumed?

1. The grid-moving mechanism has been energized.
2. The grid is moving smoothly with no jerky motions.
3. The time of the exposure is neither too short nor too long.
4. The grid table is level and parallel to the plane of the film.

5. The grid radius has been adhered to.
6. The x-ray tube is centered to the midline of the table.
7. The grid has been correctly positioned under the tabletop, with the tube side facing the x-ray tube.
8. The grid was not damaged in installation.

In the relative use of 60 to 80 kvp in medical radiography, what conversion factors are utilized in increasing the kilovoltage 10 kvp, 13 kvp, 15 kvp, and 20 kvp?

Increase 10 kvp requires a reduction to one half the mas.
Increase 13 kvp requires a reduction to one third the mas.
Increase 15 kvp requires a reduction to one fourth the mas.
Increase 20 kvp requires a reduction to one fifth the mas.

What features and uses of various grid ratios would you consider in the selection of a grid?

Table 1 may prove of assistance in the selection of a grid.

The selection of a grid is dependent upon what conditions?

The selection of a grid is dependent upon the following conditions:
1. The relative quantity of secondary radiation produced by the subject being radiographed. The quantity of secondary radiation produced is dependent on the thickness and relative density of the body part being radiographed. A nongrid exposure of the chest will consist of about one half secondary radiation, whereas a nongrid exposure of the abdomen may consist of more than 90 percent secondary radiation. It therefore is apparent that for dense body parts the more effective remover of secondary radiation will provide the most striking improvement in the radiograph.
2. The kilovoltage technique that will be used in making the radiograph at kilovoltages of the order of 100 kvp or more. Comparable photographic effect requires lower milliampere-seconds values than at low kilovoltages,

Table 1. Selecting a grid

Type	Features and uses
5:1 ratio, linear	Moderate cleanup. Extreme latitude in use. Use at lower kilovoltages (up to 80 kvp) wherever wide latitude is desired. Very easy to use.
5:1 ratio, crossed	Very high cleanup, especially at lower kilovoltages. Extreme latitude in use. Use up to 100 kvp wherever wide latitude and excellent cleanup are desired. Very easy to use. Not recommended for tilted-tube techniques.
6:1 ratio, linear	Moderate cleanup. Good positioning latitude. Easy to use.
8:1 ratio, linear	Better cleanup than 5:1 linear. Fair distance latitude. Little centering and leveling latitude. Use up to 100 kvp where wide latitude is not required.
8:1 ratio, crossed	Extremely high cleanup. Superior to 16:1 ratio, linear grid at kilovoltages up to 125. Positioning latitude equivalent to 8:1 ratio, linear. Not usable for tilted-tube techniques.
12:1 ratio, linear	Better cleanup than 8:1. Very little positioning latitude. Use for both low and high kilovoltage technique (up to 110 kvp or slightly higher). Extra care required for proper alignment in use. Usually used in fixed mount or Potter-Bucky diaphragm.
16:1 ratio, linear	Very high cleanup. Practically no positioning latitude. Intended primarily for use above 100 kvp in Potter-Bucky diaphragm. Excellent for high kv radiographs of thick body sections.

thus reducing the radiation dosage to the patient.

3. The capacity of the x-ray generator used. All technologists must work within the limitations of the physical characteristics of the x-ray equipment at their disposal. For instance, the maximum benefits to be derived from a 16:1 ratio grid will not be realized with a unit whose top limit is 90 kvp. In general, a 16:1 ratio grid will do the most good with equipment that can be used at kilovoltages above 100 kvp.

12 CONTRAST MEDIA

Contrast media or materials have been defined as substances that may be safely injected or ingested into the body tissues or organs, causing them to become visible by means of an x-ray examination. They are used in radiology as a diagnostic aid to the physician to enable him to establish the presence or absence of disease within the body. Different tissues, organs, and bones absorb radiation in varying amounts and are not always visible unless some material is used to cause them to absorb more radiation or unless surrounding tissues are made more dense, consequently making the area of interest less dense and therefore visible. All media used for x-ray examinations either will or will not inhibit the passage of x-rays through the body. Contrast media are divided into two classes. One class, including air or carbon dioxide, produces a shadow that is less dense than the surrounding structures. These materials are considered negative contrast media. The other class, including sodium iodide, produces a shadow or causes the structure of interest to be more dense than the surrounding structures. These materials are considered as positive contrast media.

Both types are used, but the positive contrast media receive more varied and frequent use. The ability of any positive contrast medium to produce a diagnostic shadow on x-ray film depends on the presence of elements in its chemical structure capable of absorbing x-rays to an extent greater than can the soft tissue structures of the body. Iodine is the most extensively used radiopaque element at the present time.

In addition to radiopacity, a contrast medium must also possess high water solubility so that it is instantly miscible with the blood and body fluids. It is essential that the viscosity of the solution be as low as possible to facilitate rapid administration; it should also be stable, easily sterilized, and inexpensive.

Any contrast medium may cause or create reactions, and for this reason histories of any allergies must be obtained prior to administering any materials. It has been stated that most reactions are minor, but, to quote an unnamed author, "Reactions are minor to all but the patient experiencing them."

Nausea, vomiting, hypotension, sweating, weakness, and urticaria are probably the most common "minor" reactions. There are numerous means of testing for sensitivity, and probably the most accurate is the injection of 1 ml. and a wait of one to three minutes before proceeding. Any reactions will probably occur during this time interval. Emergency trays should always be present and available with supplies to counteract reactions.

Constant vigilance and an awareness that each use of contrast medium is a potentially hazardous procedure is of paramount importance in the performance of the examination.

Positive contrast materials are divided into four physical states. What are they?

Positive contrast materials are those materials that absorb radiation in such quantities as to render them more dense than the surrounding tissues. They are oils, liquids, tablets, and powders.

Give a brief example of the types of materials and the examinations in which they are used.

Each of the following four materials have been found to be most effective in demonstrating certain organs and areas of the body to best advantage and causing little or no untoward reactions to the organ itself:

Material
1. Oil—Pantopaque; Dionosil
2. Liquids—Hypaque, Angio-Conray
3. Tablets—Priodex
4. Barium sulfate—Gastrografin

Organ
Myelograms, bronchograms
Pyelograms, arteriograms, angiograms
Gallbladders
Gastrointestinal—large bowel series

What are some of the important factors related to the viscosity of a contrast medium that substantiate its usage?

All reasons for using any contrast medium should fall into the category of being harmless to the patient and satisfactory for visualizing the desired area. It should also have the ability to outline mucosal patterns, be of such a viscosity that it may be injected rapidly, and have the ability to outline small bronchi but not alveoli.

On what does the opacity of any contrast material depend to a major extent?

The atomic number of the chemical mixture or compound determines the opacity of a contrast material. As the atomic number increases, the density and the ability of the medium to absorb radiation and be radiographed increases. In addition to being radiopaque, the solution also must be easily soluble.

Are radiopaque water-soluble contrast materials safe to use?

All radiopaque materials that are water soluble have been tested and found safe for intravenous use. They must be manufactured so that they are rapidly and innoculously absorbed into the blood and body tissues.

Most contrast materials have iodine content that may cause reactions. What is a danger sign that a patient might be having a reaction?

Several indications that could be noticed and acted upon rapidly are nausea, vomiting, itching of the throat, difficulty in breathing, or hives, which would show up as red blotches or welts on the face, throat, or chest. Hives are very annoying to the patient, as are most reactions.

The viscosity of contrast materials should be such that they may be injected rapidly. Is this an indication that they must be?

Definitely not. A definite correlation has been found between the frequency of reactions and the speed of injection. The faster the injection, the greater the number of reactions. All contrast agents should be injected slowly. The ideal form of examining is of course to prevent reactions, and it is toward this end that premedication with antihistamines has come into usage.

Should contrast materials be administered to patients with histories of allergies and asthma?

While allergies and asthma have frequently and loosely been considered the etiologic bases of reactions to contrast agents, there is no valid evidence that true allergy accounts for all or even the majority of reactions. In patients suffering from asthma, if indications warrant the examination being performed, then premedication with an antihistamine agent is desirable.

What procedures should you follow if you notice a patient having a reaction to an injection of contrast media?

If the reaction occurs during the injection of material, the emergency tray should be accessible to the physician so that he can administer the countersolution. If a reaction occurs after injection and the physician has left the room, the technologist should immediately notify the physician while someone stays with the patient. As stated previously, an emergency tray should be available.

What items are recommended for the emergency tray?

All emergency trays should contain: (1) airway, (2) tongue blades, (3) epinephrine, 1:1,000 aqueous solution, (4) Solu-Cortef, (5) Benadryl, (6) aminophylline, (7) amobarbital sodium, (8) phenylephrine hydrochloride, (9) levarterenol for blood pressure, and (10) syringes and needles for administering these solutions.

What contrast materials are used to visualize the gastrointestinal tract?

The contrast medium generally used is a form of barium sulfate. Barium sulfate has been found to be safe and causes no irritation to the mucosal patterns. Sulfates (barium) have been modified and micronized through various stages and for specific purposes. Changes have been made to cause them to remain in suspension for longer periods of time and to allow them to adhere to the walls of the organs being

examined. Sulfates are not to be administered when perforations are suspected because they will cause irritation and even death if allowed to enter the surrounding tissues and bloodstream.

Are all contrast materials iodine based?

Contrast materials that are to be injected intravenously are iodine based because of their ability to absorb radiation. Others are water based and therefore are not as toxic as the iodine-based media. Still others such as barium sulfate are entirely different, but they are administered orally or rectally.

For what purposes is Adrenalin used?

Adrenalin is probably the most valuable and useful drug for emergency use. It is used principally to relieve reactions caused by the injection of contrast media containing iodine. Because of its chemical composition, it will act more rapidly in relieving these reactions.

Before performing intravenous pyelograms, why should you obtain the history of a patient concerning his susceptibility or allergies?

Patients should always be questioned regarding history of allergies or asthma before injections are made. If in doubt about the information obtained from the patient, a test dose should be given prior to the injection, otherwise the chances of serious consequences occurring are magnified. While there is no clear proof that people with allergies will have reactions, it is better to take precautionary measures than to endanger the life of a patient.

Why would ginger ale or other soft drinks be used during examinations of the gastrointestinal tract?

Occasionally it is desirable to create a negative contrast (shadow) in the stomach during the examination by having gas or air present. Ginger ale will cause gas or air pockets to form because of the carbonation in its composition.

When examining a patient for the gastrointestinal area and a perforation is suspected, what media would be used and why?

It is best to use a medium with an oil base rather than barium sulfate. The material commonly used is Gastrografin, which has an oil base and because of its composition is gentle to the membranes and tissues if leaked into the tissues.

When examining the gallbladder, what type of contrast medium is used?

As with any type of examination, the patient's condition usually dictates the material used. If the patient has symptoms of pain and discomfort and if it is suspected that he has stones, the patient is given tablets the evening before the examination. The tablets are composed of chemicals that are absorbed by the gallbladder and cause it to become radiopaque. If, on the other hand, the patient is jaundiced, tablets are not administered, but a solution in liquid form would be injected that would help visualize the gallbladder after collecting there. This liquid is absorbed from the bloodstream into the gallbladder and biliary ducts, causing them to become visible. The patient's physician makes the decision as to the type of material to be used for the examination. If contrast materials are taken orally, there is usually little or no reaction, but, if the liquid type is injected, then precautions should be taken as with any other injection of a contrast medium.

What are the basic differences between intravenous cholangiograms and operative cholangiograms? What is the contrast medium used in each type of examination?

Intravenous cholangiograms are performed by injecting Cholografin into the bloodstream, from which it is absorbed by the gallbladder and pooled. Operative cholangiography is performed in the operating room or, if as a T-tube examination, perhaps in the radiology department. The gallbladder has been removed, and the injection is made either directly into the ducts or into a tube that has been inserted into the ducts. The material used is normally any radiopaque urographic medium that will be readily absorbed by the body tissues.

It has been noted that contrast materials are divided into both negative and positive contrast materials. How can you determine which have been used when viewing a finished radiograph?

Negative contrast materials, such as air or gas, allow radiation to penetrate easily and will therefore show up as dark areas on the radiograph, whereas the absorption properties of a positive contrast medium will allow it to appear white against surrounding tissues.

Why is a gas such as carbon dioxide preferred over air when doing retroperitoneal insufflations?

They are both negative contrast media and will absorb radiation to the same degree, which is very minor, but the air will cause a greater amount of irritation to the tissues than will the carbon dioxide. The carbon dioxide is less irritating, and it is absorbed more quickly by the tissues than air.

Are there examinations that may be performed using both positive and negative contrast materials, either singly or together?

There are several examinations that may be performed using both types of contrast media. Both types are useful in some examinations of the gastrointestinal tract, such as large colon, arthrograms, cystograms, and myelograms. The negative materials, being lighter than spinal fluid or other fluids, will rise, whereas the positive materials are heavier and will sink.

When would a barium examination not be performed on a patient?

If a patient were suspected of having acute appendicitis or an impaction of the lower colon, a barium examination should not be performed. The chemical composition of the barium sulfate would irritate the appendicitis and cause complications. If impaction were the diagnosis and it could not be visualized otherwise, a small amount of another contrast material could be given rectally to localize the site of impaction. If barium must be used, it should be of a consistency that will not cause additional impaction.

What material is used for myelography?

Either air or an oil may be used to visualize the spinal canal. Oil (Pantopaque) is normally used because of its atomic number and its ability to absorb radiation and thus be seen easily. It is heavier than the spinal fluid and will settle to the lower portion of the canal and follow any contour of the canal, thereby outlining any defects that may be present. It can be caused to flow from one area to another by changing the angle of the body, with the oil demonstrating the entire spinal canal. Myelography is usually performed to demonstrate any defects in the contour of the canal as a result of tumors or pathologic conditions.

What types of contrast material are used to visualize the bronchi?

Two basic types are used to demonstrate the bronchi of the lungs. They are of the oily or aqueous types. The oily type is not used too often since its properties of irritation to the lining of the lungs is greater than the aqueous type. The aqueous type, while it too is irritating, does not cause as much discomfort and may be absorbed by the tissues without harmful effects. The patient usually has the throat area anesthetized prior to beginning the examination to reduce the incidence of irritation.

Is it important that patients scheduled for examinations using contrast media refrain from eating and drinking prior to the time of the examination?

It is important that patients abstain from food and drink prior to the examination. The type of examination and the contrast media to be used will dictate the correct amount of time necessary for abstinence. This is necessary because of the possibility of causing overlying shadows or areas of increased density, which could interfere with obtaining a satisfactory examination. An examination that is not satisfactory because of interfering shadows could require rescheduling the time of the procedure.

When and if reactions to a contrast medium occur, do they do so within a specific period of time?

This is one of the reasons for administering test doses if in doubt about the patient's history. Often the reaction will occur after injection of a small, 1-ml. test dose; if not then, the indications that no reaction will occur are increased. There have been incidences in which reactions did not occur prior to, or during, examination, but did occur half an hour or even longer after injection.

List some of the earliest types of contrast media used.

In 1896, two Austrians, Haschek and Linderthal, injected a chalk-containing solution into the arterial system; Sicard and Forestier in 1923 used iodized poppyseed oil; Berberick and Hirsch in 1923 injected strontium bromide; Tineff and Stoppani in 1934 used thorium dioxide; and Fischer in 1959 used tin oxide, to name a few. Chemists have been and still are working feverishly in trying to perfect materials that will radiograph well and be tolerated by the patient.

Are technologists allowed to give injections of contrast media to patients?

There has been much discussion over the validity of this question, and, after hearing numerous experts on forensic medicine, we are still rather confused. Normally, persons administering injections should be qualified to practice medicine. Orders specifically given by a physician to give injections in no way relieves a person from the moral responsibility involved. We will state that technologists should not administer injections since serious consequences may result if a fatal reaction were to occur.

13 PEDIATRIC RADIOGRAPHY

Pediatric radiography is the term used in describing radiographs of infants and children. Of course, changes are necessary when dealing with infants and children because of the changes in composition of the bones and the soft tissue. Not only are the anatomic changes a consideration, but children, when placed in strange surroundings, are apprehensive and frightened and require additional tact and ingenuity on the part of the technologist. The utmost tact and ingenuity are necessary to assure satisfactory radiographs when the patient is crying, moving, or being generally uncooperative. This situation is often the case when dealing with children and infants. Because of their ages, additional precautions must be taken to assure a reduction in the amount of radiation received by the patient. Exposure should always be reduced to a minimum, but, when dealing with infants, it is even more important. Until recently, pediatrics was a part of general radiography, but, because of the need for special handling, it has evolved into a separate specialty and, because it has assumed this position, is resulting in a better method of obtaining satisfactory radiographs in infants and children.

Why do radiographic examinations of infants differ from those of adults?

The infant's skeletal system has not developed and must be radiographed using a completely different set of technical factors. The child is often too young to understand what is being done and what is expected of him and therefore lacks the ability to cooperate and suspend respiration. The strange department and people cause the infant to become apprehensive and frightened. His fright causes him to react in a manner that he understands and is familiar with to get relief and satisfaction.

When dealing with infants, what are some standards that should be observed to assure radiographic consistency?

A suitable standard technique should be followed using either the variable kvp technique or the fixed kvp technique. Whatever the technique, it should be observed. Restraining and immobilizing equipment should be available and utilized constantly. When observing these procedures and standard processing, it will be found that consistent radiographs will be obtainable.

Projections often vary for radiographs of infants and adults. What are some of the differences when radiographing the dorsal and lumbar vertebrae?

Radiographs of the dorsal and lumbar vertebrae in infants are usually performed

134

using one film, which will cover both areas in the anteroposterior projection, utilizing correct coning and protective shielding. An additional projection (lateral), done with proper protection and coning, is also taken, again utilizing one film to demonstrate both the dorsal and lumbar spines. When radiographing adults for the dorsal and lumbar areas, each area is radiographed separately. The dorsal spine is radiographed in the anteroposterior and lateral projections, each projection using a separate film, coning, and shielding. The same procedure is used for the lumbar area. For infants two films are utilized for anteroposterior and lateral projections of the dorsal and lumbar spines, whereas in adults four films are used, two for the dorsal and two for the lumbar areas.

Restraining bands preferably should be of what types of material?

Restraining bands should be made of a translucent material that will not interfere with the resultant radiograph. When radiographing infants, it has been found that plastic or transparent restraints are beneficial since using them will allow observation of the body part being restrained. In observing the body one can visualize the correct positioning of the body and correctly place the part to the film and cone.

In pediatric radiology, when changing from a Bucky exposure to a non-Bucky exposure, what basic rules are followed?

Because of the construction, or formation, of the infant's anatomy and bony structure, changes are required. We know that the exposure must be less because of the inability of the bones to absorb radiation. It has been found that when converting techniques from Bucky to non-Bucky the milliampere-seconds must be reduced by one half and the kilovoltage reduced by five. This will assure a radiograph of a satisfactory diagnostic quality.

Why is it important that instructions and emergency equipment be available when doing excretory urography on children?

The technician should be familiar with the use of all emergency equipment and should have it readily available for immediate use in the event that it is needed. When radiographing infants, unless a parent is present, there is no satisfactory method of obtaining a history of allergy or other symptoms that might cause reactions. Even with parents' answers to questions there is always the possibility of a reaction, and emergency equipment must be present.

Why is it advantageous to have and use rapid timers when doing pediatric radiography?

Motion is a major reason for repeating examinations, especially when doing infants. Repeats are to be condemned because of the increase in radiation to the patient. Infants are apprehensive and frightened, and speed is of vital importance. To be able to select a time that will stop motion is desirable. Even using rapid timers, the technician is required to synchronize the exposure to the respirations of the patient to suspend or stop motion. Rapid impulse timers make this feat possible.

Why is preparing the room, technique, film, and other equipment prior to bringing the patient into the room important?

Apprehension in infants of different ages is likely to vary, and they might cause themselves bodily harm, such as bumping their heads, banging their feet, or rolling off the table onto the floor, causing untold damage. If the technologist has the room, technique, and films ready, then the dangers are reduced and the results improved.

Why, when radiographing extremities on infants, are both sides done?

Both extremities should be radiographed because of the growth of bones and the time element involved. Since there is a definite relationship between the infant's age and the bone growth that has taken place, it is beneficial to radiograph both extremities so that any abnormal growth patterns may be recognized by comparison.

When radiographing an infant's skull in the lateral projection, where should the central ray be positioned?

The skull should be immobilized in the true lateral position by using positioning blocks and a plastic restraining band. The orbital, or acanthomeatal, line should be parallel to the tabletop, and the central ray should be perpendicular to the film and centered to enter the skull 1½ inches superior to the acanthomeatal line and midway between the outer canthus of the eye and the external auditory canal. The exposure should be made when movement has ceased, if it is present.

Which examination carries the possibility of the greatest exposure to the patient?

Unless protective measures are adequately utilized, all examinations, especially those covering the reproductive areas, are potentially hazardous. During fluoroscopy of the gastrointestinal tract, the greatest potential of excessive radiation is realized since protective devices cannot be adequately utilized because of the nature of the examination. Every precaution is taken to assure that the smallest amount of radiation is received by the patient.

How may exposure to personnel be reduced during fluoroscopy?

The primary objective of equipment manufacturers today is to reduce radiation to both the patient and the employee or operator. During fluoroscopy it is necessary that the operator be close to the fluoroscope to adequately perform the examination, and because of this requirement, shutters are incorporated over the tube to restrict the field size. Lead aprons

and gloves, which should be worn by the operator, lead shields attached to the fluoroscope, image amplification, and remote control viewing are methods of reducing the radiation. High kilovoltage at short times and restraining devices also should be used.

Why is it advantageous to radiograph infants in the x-ray department, as opposed to doing portable examinations?

Radiography in the x-ray department is preferred because of the desire to reduce radiation to a minimum. Also, the equipment, restraining devices, positioning aids, and other equipment are available in the department and are not on the wards. It is not feasible to move all necessary devices to the wards when doing portables; therefore, not only does the patient usually receive more radiation but also, because of the lack of aids, the results are not always satisfactory, which often necessitates repeats. The medical staff should be made aware of these reasons, and, if they are properly informed, the number of requests for portable examinations will be reduced. The results will be better diagnosis, less radiation to the patient, and generally a better relationship between staff physicians, nurses, and radiologists.

Why are parents asked not to accompany the child into the radiographic examining room?

Parents are asked not to accompany children primarily because, as parents, they are emotionally involved and are prone to believe that the child is being harmed because of his crying, kicking, and screaming. If they are present, they tend to console the child, and this interferes with the technician's performance of his duties. The technician should be able to cope with the situation and usually can if the parents are not present. The presence of the parent often causes the child to react even more.

Why is it not mandatory that children scheduled for barium enemas be cleansed by taking castor oil the night before the examination?

Because of the physiology of the infant, the food ingested does not create overlying objectional shadows, and the abnormalities found in children are not obscured by the lack of preparation, except possibly in the event of polyps in the colon. If the possibility of polyps exists, then it might require the administering of castor oil or some other cathartic to assist in cleansing the colon as completely as possible. Because of the nature of polyps, to demonstrate them all overlying shadows should be removed or every possible effort should be exerted to assure that there will be no objectional gas or feces.

Why would a child scheduled for a barium enema who suffers from Hirschsprung's disease not be filled completely during the examination?

Hirschsprung's disease is a congenital hypertrophic dilation of the colon, and patients suffering from it are unable to evacuate properly. Because of this inability to evacuate, it would be extremely unwise to fill the colon completely since serious impaction could occur. The examination should never create a situation that will increase the dangers from the disease.

Are children between 2 and 5 years of age usually able to understand what is required of them when they are requested to cooperate?

This is a debatable question, and no specific answer will suffice since each child must be evaluated individually and treated accordingly. Some children in this age group are able to understand and cooperate, and others will if the technologist will take the time and patience to explain what is required. Children, like adults, respond to patience and understanding and must be treated individually, not grouped together. The technologist has to be able to evaluate each case as to the child's maturity and emotional state and make a decision from his observations. There will be those children in this age bracket on which nothing one says or does will have any effect; these then require a different approach and tact.

Why would nonelastic restraining bands or bandages be used rather than the elastic types?

Whenever any bandages or restraining bands are used, they should be of a type that are nonradiopaque and will not show on the radiographs. Any foreign object used will be radiographed and will interfere with the resultant radiograph. Nonelastic bandages contain no materials that will show on the radiograph and therefore are desirable, whereas elastic bandages contain rubber that will show on the radiograph and are therefore objectionable.

When radiographing children for acute abdominal pain, how many views are usually taken?

Unlike adult radiography, in which the patient is able to describe the pain, children are usually unable to adequately describe their symptoms. Adults have an anteroposterior recumbent view of the abdomen and, if able to stand, an erect anteroposterior view to show any air or fluid that might be present in the abdominal cavity. Children usually require three views—anteroposterior, recumbent, and lateral. Often special views are required to demonstrate some pathologic conditions. In cases of imperforate anus, inverted abdomen films are taken.

When radiographing mastoids and sinuses in infants, what projections are taken?

The views taken to demonstrate the paranasal sinuses are the anteroposterior projection, reverse Waters, and lateral projection. In the anteroposterior projection the infant is wrapped securely in Ace bandages for purposes of immobilization. The infant is placed on his back, and the central ray is centered to the midline slightly above the root of the nose. Projections for the mastoids are the Chamberlain-Towne and Law projections of each mastoid. In the anteroposterior projection of Chamberlain-Towne the central ray is centered to the midline at the level of the hairline, with the tube angled 30 to 35 degrees toward the feet. In the Law projection the patient is positioned as for a lateral skull, with the affected side nearest the film and the tube angled 15 degrees toward the feet and 15 degrees toward the face.

When occasion warrants doing special radiographic studies, pneumoencephalography and ventriculography of the skull in infants, what views are taken?

When doing any of these studies, the infant is wrapped from the shoulders down to the feet in Ace bandages to minimize motion, and the views taken are anteroposterior, Chamberlain-Towne, brow-up lateral, right lateral, left lateral, posteroanterior, brow-down, reverse modified Chamberlain-Towne, and, if studying hydrocephalies, an inverted or upside-down lateral.

What projections are used to radiograph the scapula in children?

The views used in radiography of the scapula are the anteroposterior and lateral projections. Positioning for the anteroposterior scapula is the same as that for a view of the shoulder. The lateral projection is performed with the child in the anterior oblique position, with the side of interest against the table. The central ray is directed slightly medial to the vertebral border of the scapula at the level of the shoulder joint.

What views are taken to demonstrate ribs above and below the diaphragm?

The routine views taken to demonstrate ribs on children are the anteroposterior, left posterior oblique, right posterior oblique, and posteroanterior projections. In the event of injury to the anterior portions of the chest, anterior oblique films, both left and right, are taken in place of the posterior obliques. Except for larger children, it is unnecessary to make separate exposures for the ribs above and below the diaphragm since all ribs will be satisfactorily demonstrated on the routine films.

What views are taken to demonstrate the sternum?

The routine views are right and left anterior oblique projections of the thorax and Pancoast lateral of the chest. The oblique views are exposed using Bucky technique, whereas the Pancoast lateral projection has the child sitting with one side against the cassette and both arms pulled behind the body, with the chin elevated slightly. The Pancoast lateral projection requires about 5 kvp more than the lateral chest technique.

What are the routine views taken for facial bones?

The routine views are posteroanterior, Waters, 30-degree Waters, lateral, both laterals of the nasal bones, and occlusal projection of the nasal bones. The posteroanterior projection is positioned as for the skull. The Waters projection has the central ray directed to the midline at the vertex and through the root of the nose; the 30-degree Waters projection has the central ray directed to the midline at the vertex, with the tube angled 30 degrees caudad and projected through the inferior orbital margin. In lateral views the central ray is directed to the zygomatic bone nearest the tube; occlusal view has the central ray directed horizontal to the film along the midline tangential to the forehead.

What, if any, are the differences between

children and adult projections when examining the gastrointestinal tract?

During gastrointestinal studies in adults, they are fluoroscoped and spot films are taken; after fluoroscopy routine posteroanterior, right anterior oblique, right lateral, and anteroposterior views are taken. In children the procedure is almost the same except that, after spot films are taken during fluoroscopy, the next film taken is an anteroposterior projection of the abdomen fifteen to thirty minutes after fluoroscopy.

Are there special urographic contrast agents used for infants and children?

Special contrast agents are not generally used, but discretion must be exercised in the selection. Any urographic opacifying agent can be used in comparable dosages. Any solution of 50 percent or higher concentrations cannot be used for intramuscular injections because of the risk of serious local reactions with resultant tissue necrosis and breakdown. If intramuscular injections are necessary, solutions of 35 percent concentration should be used.

What views and procedures are followed for myelography?

When performing myelography in children, preliminary anteroposterior and lateral projections are taken of the vertebral column of interest. Spot films are taken during fluoroscopy of the vertebral column and any specific areas of pathology. Posteroanterior, lateral cross table projections of the vertebral column, with the column of dye at the level of the suspected pathologic alteration and anteroposterior projection of the vertebral column, and lateral projection of the skull are taken after the contrast material has been removed from the subarachnoid space.

When we refer to growth study in pediatrics, to what do we refer?

Growth study is a study of the measurements of the length of the lower extremities by direct measurement of the radiographic bone length. Occasionally the upper extremities are measured.

What is a scoliosis study?

A scoliosis study is the radiographic analysis of abnormal spinal curvatures for mobility, correctability, and structural change prior to, and during, orthopedic treatment.

REFERENCE

Darling, D. B.: Radiography in infants and children, Springfield, Ill., 1962, Charles C Thomas, Publisher.

14 DENTAL RADIOGRAPHY

Dental radiography, like any other area of examination, requires a thorough knowledge of the structures and anatomy of the teeth. Positioning requires accurate placement of both the film and the tube to assure the best detail and visible results. Too much or too little angulation can result in an elongated or foreshortened image of the teeth.

How many sets of teeth are there?

There are two sets of teeth: the temporary, or deciduous, and the permanent.

How many teeth are in each set?

The deciduous teeth are twenty in number and are usually seen between the ages of six months and three years. There are thirty-two permanent teeth. They usually replace the temporary teeth between the sixth and the twenty-first year.

Are the teeth divided into any particular order for each jaw?

Yes. In adults there are sixteen teeth in each jaw, with the jaw being divided into an upper and lower section.

What are the teeth called in each jaw?

The sixteen teeth in each jaw are called incisors, cuspids, bicuspids, and molars.

How many of each teeth are there in each jaw?

There are four incisors, two cuspids, four bicuspids, and six molars. The two posterior molars are called wisdom teeth.

What is the part of the jaw called that contains the teeth?

This part of the jaw is called the alveolar process. Both the maxilla and the mandible have alveolar processes.

What are the main parts of a tooth?

Each tooth has three main parts: the root, the neck, and the crown.

Briefly describe the tooth in relation to the alveolar process.

The root of the tooth is embedded in the alveolar process and is covered with a substance called cement. The neck of the tooth is located between the root and the gum line.

Where is the crown of the tooth located?

The crown is located above the gum line and is the area of the tooth visible to the eye.

How is a tooth structured?

From the inside to the outside the tooth contains a pulp cavity, which extends from the crown through the root, ending at a small opening at the apex of the root called the foramen. Surrounding the pulp cavity is modified bone called the dentin;

covering the dentin of the root is a layer of modified bone called the cementum. The periodontal membrane is a fibrous membrane lying between the cementum of the root and the adjacent surrounding bone. The neck of the tooth is protected by the dentin, whereas the crown is protected by enamel.

Because of the structure and shape of the teeth, the surface areas have been given different names. What are they?

There are five basic surfaces to each tooth. They are listed as follows:

Occlusal. The biting surface or the surface on the bicuspids and molars used for chewing. It is known as the "incisal edge" on incisors and cuspids.

Buccal. The surface of the tooth facing the cheeks or lips or bicuspids and molars. On the incisors and cuspids it is known as the "labial surface." It is sometimes referred to as "facial" for all teeth.

Lingual. That surface near or closest to the tongue on all teeth.

Medial. The surface contacting adjacent teeth in the same arch. Those teeth closest to the midline are termed medial.

Distal. The surface away from the midline and toward the back of the mouth.

The crown of the tooth is covered by enamel. What is enamel?

Enamel is a very dense, whitish substance around (outside) the dentin and covering the crown of the tooth. It is the hardest substance in the body and appears radiopaque on a radiograph. It is inert.

What is dentin?

Dentin is the layer under the enamel. Unlike the enamel, which is inert, dentin is alive and will form new dentin if necessary to protect the nerves in the pulp. It is yellow in color and is not as dense as enamel.

What is the purpose of the pulp?

The pulp contains the nerve and blood supply for the tooth. When contacted or exposed to direct contact with hot or cold solutions it will respond as "pain." It is the central portion of a tooth and is covered by the cementum, which is a thin layer and is barely discernible on a radiograph.

Where is the periodontal membrane?

The periodontal membrane surrounds each tooth, acting as a ligament to support the tooth within its bony socket. It is radiolucent. It also contains cells, blood vessels, and nerves responsible for the sensation of touch when chewing or clenching.

How many roots are there to the tooth?

The incisors, cuspids, upper second bicuspids, and lower first and second bicuspids have one root each. The lower molars have two roots: a mesial and a distal. The upper molars have three roots: one distobuccal, one mesiobuccal, and one lingual.

When radiographing the teeth, how are they identified?

There are two methods employed, the Palmer and the numerical. The different notations are both based on looking directly into the patient's face.

What are the differences between the two?

The Palmer method divides the face (teeth) into upper, lower, right, and left quadrants, listed from the right, as follows:

$$R \quad \frac{87654321 \mid 12345678}{87654321 \mid 12345678}$$

Teeth are distinguished by number and by position of the lines. For example, 8| means right upper third molar; |8 means left lower third molar.

The numerical system lists as follows:

$$R\ \frac{1\ 2\ 3\ 4\ 5\ 6\ 7\ 8}{32\ 31\ 30\ 29\ 28\ 27\ 26\ 25}\ \bigg|\ \frac{9\ 10\ 11\ 12\ 13\ 14\ 15\ 16}{24\ 23\ 22\ 21\ 20\ 19\ 18\ 17}$$

What differences, if any, exist between deciduous teeth and permanent teeth?

The deciduous teeth are smaller, more bell-shaped, and whiter and have more flared roots. They are also fewer in number. There are no deciduous bicuspids so that the deciduous first molars are found directly distal to the deciduous cuspids.

What are the muscles of mastication?

The muscles of mastication are those muscles that through their contraction control the opening and closing of the jaws. They apply a force acting through the teeth of the mandibular dental arch against the teeth of the maxillary dental arch during the various movements of mastication. The muscles are (1) masseter, (2) temporal, (3) external pterygoid, and (4) internal pterygoid. The external pterygoids aid in depressing the mandible by drawing the condyles forward.

Once the mouth is open, how does it remain open, since the muscles of mastication are acting to force it closed?

The suprahyoid muscles hold the chin down and resist the forward drift, thus tilting the body of the mandible. The suprahyoid and infrahyoid muscles also assert some control over the act of mastication through their activity in applying counterforces to those greater forces that are brought to bear by the more powerful muscles of mastication. They come into play during extreme depression of the mandible during lateral movement of the mandible beyond the functional movements of mastication, when the mouth is opened at its widest.

Where is the buccinator muscle located, and what is its function?

The buccinator muscle belongs to the group of muscles controlling facial expressions. It is located in the cheek and functions with the tongue in the placement of food between the teeth during mastication.

Where are the muscles of mastication located?

The masseter muscle, a flat, quadrangular muscle, has an origin that is partly tendinous and partly fleshy. It arises in two parts: superficially from the lower border of the zygomatic arch in its anterior two thirds, and more deeply from the deep surface of the zygomatic arch in its whole length. It is partially concealed by the parotid gland. It conceals the ramus of the mandible.

The temporal muscle is fan-shaped, arising from the whole of the temporal fossa and from the temporal fascia. Its converging fibers form a thick tendon as they pass medial to the zygomatic arch. Its lower fibers become continuous with the buccinator muscle.

The lateral pterygoid muscle is deeply placed in the infratemporal fossa. It arises by two heads, upper and lower. The upper head is attached to the infratemporal surface of the greater wing of the sphenoid; the lower head originates from the lateral surface of the lateral pterygoid plate. The muscle is directed laterally and backward to be inserted into the front of the neck of the mandible.

The internal pterygoid has a double origin: (1) from the medial surface of the lateral pterygoid plate and the posterior surface of the tubercle of the palatine bone, and (2) from the tuberosity of the maxilla. It is quadrilateral in form and is directed downward, laterally, and backward to be inserted into a triangular impression on the medial surface of the mandible.

Is there a nerve supply to the facial muscles? If so, which nerves?

All of the muscles of mastication are supplied with nerves. The mandibular division of the trigeminal nerve supplies all the muscles of mastication. The internal pterygoid is supplied by the nerve before it divides; all others are supplied by the anterior division.

What are nutrient canals?

Nutrient canals contain blood vessels and nerves that supply the teeth, interdental spaces, and gingivae. They appear as radiolucent lines of rather uniform width on the radiograph. The nutrient canals of the mandible are more often visualized than those of the maxilla. The nutrient canals vary greatly in size and in location in relation to the roots of the teeth.

The interdental canals are often seen in the anterior regions of the mandible, especially in cases in which the alveolar process is very thin. In some instances foramina from which branches emerge to the external surfaces of the maxilla may be seen as small radiolucent areas between and at about the level of the root apexes of the teeth.

There are ridges, processes, and tubercles visualized on the radiograph taken of the dental arches; what are they?

One structure appearing radiopaque on a radiograph is the external oblique ridge, which is a continuation of the anterior border of the ramus as it passes forward and downward over the outer surface of the body of the mandible to the mental ridge. The mylohyoid ridge begins on the medial and anterior aspect of the ramus and extends downward and forward diagonally on the lingual surface of the mandible toward the lower border of the symphysis. The mental ridge is located on the anterior aspect and near the inferior border of the mandible. It extends from the premolar region to the symphysis.

The zygomatic process of the maxilla originates on the lateral surface directly above the first molar region, extending upward in varying degrees.

The coronoid process of the mandible moves forward when the mouth is opened.

The hamular process is a bony projection arising from the sphenoid bone, extending downward and slightly posterior. Its length, width, and shape vary from patient to patient.

The genial tubercles are situated on the lingual surface of the mandible about midway between the superior and inferior borders. There are four of them, two on each side adjacent to the symphysis.

What is the stylohyoid chain?

The stylohyoid chain consists of the styloid process of the temporal bone, the lesser cornu or horn of the hyoid bone, and the connection between the two. In many mammals this cartilage gives rise to a series of four bony parts, variously called tympanohyal, stylohyal, epihyal, and ceratohyal.

Define these additional terms employed in dental radiography.

labial toward the lips
buccal toward the cheek
lingual toward the tongue
mesial toward the midline
facial (includes labial and buccal) the side of the tooth toward the face
deciduous falling off; those teeth that are shed (baby teeth)
succedaneous ensuing, in place of
occlusal plane that plane determined by the occluding surfaces of the teeth

What are cusps?

Cusps are prominences on the flattened surfaces of the crown, separated by shallow grooves.

What is meant by the term "malocclusion"?

Malocclusion is a condition that exists when teeth lying opposite each other on each side do not touch.

In dental radiography what examinations are performed?

The three types of examinations in dental radiography are the periapical, for the entire tooth and its surrounding structures; the interproximal, to detect caries on the proximal surfaces; and the occlusal, to examine large areas of the maxilla or mandible for fractures, pathology, root fragments, and unerupted teeth.

What is the ala tragus line?

The ala tragus line is a line drawn from the ala of the nose to the tragus of the ear. When examing the maxillary region, this line should be horizontal to the floor.

When examining the mandibular region, is the ala tragus line still used?

No. When radiographing the mandible, the line should be drawn from the tragus of the ear to the corner of the mouth, and this line should be horizontal to the floor.

May the film be bent when inserting it into the patient's mouth?

Yes, slightly. However, it should be straightened after insertion to relieve any distortion that will result if it remains bent.

Is motion a factor to be considered when doing dental radiographs?

Motion is always a factor to be considered. Motion will cause blurring and necessitate repeats. The patient should be instructed to cooperate as much as possible by holding his head and the film still.

Are there different angulations used in dental radiography?

There are two distinct angulations used in relation to the horizontal or occlusal plane. Any angle from above the line, or plane, intersecting it is said to be plus-degree angulation; any angle, or plane, from below the horizontal is said to be minus-degree angulation.

Can either side of the dental film be used next to the tube?

No, it may not. Each dental film has an embossed dot to denote tube side, and this dot should always be nearest the tube. Lead foil is on the opposite side to clear up scatter, and if turned toward the tube will result in poor, if any, radiographs.

When the resultant radiograph shows an elongation of the teeth, what is the cause?

The central ray is directed from too low an angle through the tooth, causing elongation.

What causes a foreshortening of the image?

Central ray projection from too high an angle and bisecting the teeth will cause a foreshortening of the image.

Are there specific rules for the degree of angulation to be used?

Definitely. To reproduce an accurate image of a tooth, the central ray must be projected perpendicular to a plane bisecting the angle formed by the longitudinal axis of the tooth and the plane of the film pocket.

How does one prevent overlapping of the teeth?

By directing the central ray through the interproximal spaces of the teeth, that is, between the teeth, overlapping can be prevented.

REFERENCES

Mallett, M.: Handbook of anatomy and physiology, ed. 4, Wisconsin, 1962, The American Society of Radiologic Technology.

U. S. Navy Manual, revised 1963, Bethesda, Md., U. S. Navy Medical School, National Naval Medical Center.

X-rays in density, Rochester, N. Y., 1962, Eastman Kodak Co.

15 RADIOLOGIC PHYSICS

What is a volt?

The volt is a unit of pressure that will force 1 ampere of current through 1 ohm of resistance, or it might be stated that voltage is the potential difference between two points.

What is a kilovolt?

A kilovolt or kilovoltage is a term used to refer to the electromotive force across the tube; it determines the penetrating power of the emitted x-rays. "Kilo" denotes 1,000.

What is an ampere?

The ampere is a practical unit of measurement indicating the quantity of electrical current flowing through a conductor in one second. It has been computed that 1 ampere of current is equal to a flow of 6.25×10^{18} electrons per second, or 6.25 billion billion electrons per second.

What is a milliampere?

A milliampere is a unit of current used to measure the quantity of electrons that flow across the x-ray tube. One milliampere is equal to one thousandth of 1 ampere.

What is an ohm?

An ohm is a unit of measurement of resistance. It represents the resistance of a conductor that permits 1 ampere of current to flow through it when a pressure of 1 volt is applied to the ends of the conductor.

What are some factors that affect resistance?

1. Size of the conductor
2. Length of the conductor
3. Diameter of the conductor
4. Construction (material) of the conductor
5. Temperature of the conductor

What is an element?

An element is matter whose atoms have the same weights and physical characteristics. Examples of such are copper, hydrogen, and lead.

How are elements arranged?

All of the known elements can be arranged into a table in which they are grouped by atomic number and chemical similarities. This arrangement is known as the periodic chart of the atoms.

What is meant by substance?

Substance can be defined as any material that has a definite and constant composition.

What is a compound?

A compound is the union of two or more

elements that may be separated only by chemical means. The elements are usually of definite proportions. An example of this is salt, which contains one atom of sodium and one of chlorine.

What is an atom?

An atom is the smallest particle of matter retaining all of the chemical properties of the element. The atom is composed of protons, neutrons, and electrons.

What is a molecule?

A molecule is the smallest particle of matter that has retained all the physical and chemical properties of the original substance. The compactness of the molecules determines whether it will be a solid, liquid, or gas.

What is meant by mixture?

Mixture is the physical combination of two or more elements that may be separated by physical means. An example of a mixture is air.

Explain atomic structure.

The atom is divided into the nucleus, which contains one or more protons and neutrons, around which electrons move in an orbital shell. Protons are positively charged particles; neutrons are neutral particles, and electrons are negatively charged particles. A neutral atom has the same number of electrons in its orbits as there are protons in the nucleus.

What is meant by the mass number of the atom?

The mass number of the atom is determined by adding the number of protons and neutrons together. This is also referred to as the A number.

What is meant by atomic number?

Atomic number is designated as the number of positive charges (protons) on the atomic nucleus. This is also referred to as the Z number.

What is atomic weight?

The weight of atoms is compared to the arbitrarily assigned weight of oxygen as 16. It is approximately equal to the sum of all protons and neutrons within the nucleus.

What are nucleons?

Nucleons are particles in the nucleus, either protons or neutrons.

What is energy?

Energy is the capacity to work. There are two types of energy. Kinetic energy, which is the energy of motion, derives its meaning from the Greek word *kinetikas*. Potential energy is the energy at rest that becomes kinetic energy when put into motion.

What is binding energy of an electron?

The binding energy of an electron is the energy required to remove the particle from its orbit.

What is matter?

Matter is anything that occupies space and has weight and dimensions.

What is a watt?

The watt is a unit of power. Power is the time that work is done. The watt is equal to 10^7 ergs or 1 joule per second. One thousand watts is a kilowatt.

What was Bohr's theory of the atom?

In his theory Bohr compared atomic structure to that of a solar system in which the planets revolve around the sun. He represented the sun as the nucleus of the atom and the planets orbiting around the sun as the electrons. The maximum number of electrons in the shells is predetermined. The shells are designated by letters of the alphabet, with K being the innermost orbit.

What is Coulomb's law?

Coulomb's law states in part that like

charges repel each other and unlike charges attract each other.

What is ionization?

A charged atom, or ion, is formed by adding or removing an electron from a neutral atom. Positive ions result from the removal of electrons, whereas negative ions are the result of additional electrons. This process of converting atoms to ions is called ionization.

What methods are there for producing ionization?

Ionization may be produced by the following methods:
1. The bombardment of matter by x-ray
2. Decay or breakdown of radioactive material
3. Chemical reaction
4. Light (such as that used in the photo-electric cell)
5. Thermionic emission

What is Ohm's law?

Ohm's law states that the intensity of the current (amperes) in any conductor is equal to the difference in potential (volts) divided by the resistance (ohms). It is expressed as:

$$I = \frac{E}{R}$$

where

I = Current
E = Voltage
R = Resistance

If any two of the factors are known, the third may be found by inserting the known in the formula.

What is magnetism?

A property of certain substances to attract pieces of iron is known as magnetism.

What is a magnet?

A magnet is a substance possessing the property of attracting or repelling other substances by an invisible force. There are three types of magnets: natural magnets (such as the earth or lodestone), artificial magnets (pieces of steel that have been magnetized), and electromagnets (produced by means of an electric current).

What are the laws of magnetism?

1. Every magnet has a north and south pole.
2. Like poles repel each other, whereas unlike poles attract each other.
3. The force of attraction or repulsion between magnets varies directly with the strength of the poles and inversely with the square of the distance.

What is a magnetic field?

The magnetic field is the area about a magnet, or conductor, through which the lines of force pass.

What is an electromagnet?

An electromagnetic is a device that consists of a coil and a core, the core consisting of a magnetizable material, and that becomes a magnet when a current is sent through the coil.

Explain electromagnetic induction.

Electromagnetic induction is the process of inducing a current in a circuit as a result of changes in the electromagnetic field about a nearby circuit. The induced voltage depends upon certain factors, which include the speed of the wire cutting the magnetic field, the strength of the magnetic field, the angle with which the magnetic field is cut, and the number of turns of wire in the coil.

What is self-induction?

Self-induction is produced in a conductor when changes in current are produced by the rapid expansion and contraction of a magnetic field. When cutting across the expanding magnetic field, the decreasing magnetic field produces a counterelectromotive force.

Explain mutual induction.

Mutual induction is the production of an induced electromagnetic force in one circuit by a changing current in another. This occurs when the flux from one coil cuts across that of another. The amount of mutual induction depends upon the position of the two coils.

What is a transformer?

A transformer is a device that transfers power from one part of a circuit to another part by means of mutual induction between its primary and secondary coil. Voltage may be increased or decreased in respect to the type of transformer used. The basic principle of a transformer is based upon the theory of mutual induction.

How many types of transformers are there, and how are they constructed?

There are basically two types of transformers, a step-up and a step-down transformer. In the step-up transformer the secondary coil has more coils of wire than the primary. In the step-down the opposite is true. The basic components of a transformer are the core, which is made of a laminated steel alloy that tends to reduce transformer loss, and a primary coil, which consists of a number of turns of insulated wires and a secondary winding that receives its electromagnetic force from the primary by induction. Transformers may be open-core, closed-core, or shell type.

Autotransformers are necessary for x-ray equipment. What are they, and why are they necessary?

Autotransformers are transformers with a single winding to control high voltage. There is a direct connection between the primary and secondary coils, which also utilize the principle of self-induction.

The autotransformer is constructed by winding a coil of insulated wire around an iron core. At separate and definite intervals along the core, taps are drawn off. A con-tactor may be moved along these taps, thus varying the coils of wire utilized and varying the output voltage.

What mechanism, besides the autotransformer, is used to control high voltage?

A rheostat utilizing either direct or alternating current is used to control high voltage. The rheostat is constructed with a series of resistance coils and a method of varying the resistance. The variable resistance will produce a variable voltage.

What purpose has the choke coil in the circuit?

A choke coil is a device used for regulating current in a circuit. It consists of a coil of wire and a soft iron core that may be moved in and out of the coil. The choke coil is used to vary the current to the filament of the x-ray tube and changes the electron emission of the filament.

What is rectification?

Rectification is the conversion of alternating current to direct current. This is done by limiting, or adjusting, the direction of current flow.

The simplest form of rectification is self-rectification. We know that the current flows from cathode to anode. During the positive half of the cycle, the cathode allows the current to flow. In the negative half of the cycle, the current is flowing toward the anode. Since the anode does not produce free electrons and is not hot, the inverse voltage is stopped. Only when the anode becomes hot enough to allow free electrons to be emitted does the voltage drive the electrons to the filament.

Another means of rectification is mechanical. As modern technologists, we realize that this is obsolete.

The valve tube is another means of rectification. The valve tube rectifiers are glass envelopes, highly evacuated like an x-ray tube. They contain a filament wire made of tungsten and a metal plate like an anode. One valve tube may be used to suppress the voltage in one half of the cycle. This is called half-wave rectification. The tube is placed in series with the x-ray tube and connected so that, when the electrons flow from the valve tube filament to the anode, the electrons will also flow the same way in the x-ray tube. In the inverse cycle the anode of the tube is used to stop the flow of voltage.

If you wish to save wear and tear on the anode of the tube, another valve tube may be introduced into the circuit. This tube must also be in series with the x-ray tube and the other valve tube. Now, when the inverse phase is present, the valve tube on the anode side suppresses the flow of negative voltage. One must remember that the flow of voltage will only be in one direction and that the use of one or two valve tubes only produces half-wave rectification.

To use both phases of the voltage cycle one may use four valve tubes. Two of them are connected in series with the x-ray tube when the positive phase is utilized, and the other two are connected in series with the x-ray tube in the negative phase. When thus connected, the current will flow only into two valve tubes at one-half cycle.

What advantages does the four-valve rectification have?

In modern x-ray equipment the valve tubes are usually immersed in oil in the high-tension transformer tank, thus eliminating dangers of having any part of the high tension circuit out in the open.

By immersing the valve tubes in oil the amount of insulation built into a transformer tank is reduced. Also connections from the center tap of the transformer to ground the highest potential of any part of the circuit in relation to the ground will be one half the kilovoltage.

Since the valve tube has no moving parts, the rectification is noiseless. While immersed in oil, there will be no arcing

across as with mechanical means. Valve tubes in themselves receive little wear and tear and thus will have a long usage.

The use of four valves allows the use of higher voltages and higher currents by the technologist without danger of damaging the x-ray tube.

Why is rectified voltage needed for use in x-ray equipment?

X-ray equipment, especially the x-ray tube, operates only when the flow of electrons is from cathode to anode. While the anode is made to dissipate heat, it can become so hot with excessive and continuous exposures that it will emit electrons and thus create conductivity to the filament, resulting in tube damage. Therefore, the efficient rectification of both cycles gives a constant flow of electrons to the target.

What is thermionic emission?

Thermionic emission is the freeing of electrons in the wire by means of heat. Thermionic emission is most frequently used in electron tubes. Secondary emission can occur in the valve tubes when other electrons strike the surface of the target at high velocity and cause emissions of electrons from the body struck. Since this is undesirable, it must be controlled.

What are roentgenology and radiology?

Roentgenology is the branch of science that deals with x-rays, especially their use for diagnosis or treatment in medicine and dentistry.

Radiology is the science of x-rays and radioactive material and their application in the diagnosis and cure of disease.

Roentgenography deals with photographic recording by means of x-rays. In the beginning glass plates were used, and then photographic paper was used, until the present x-ray film was developed.

What are x-rays?

X-rays are electromagnetic waves that

travel with the speed of light, or 186,000 miles per second.

How are x-rays produced?

X-rays primarily result from the sudden change (deceleration) in the velocity of a moving electric charge, as when rapidly moving electrons strike a solid target in a vacuum tube, and as a result of changes in the target caused by this impact.

What are the properties of x-rays?

1. X-rays are electromagnetic radiation, which means that they possess characteristics similar to other types of radiation. The product of their frequency and their wavelength equals the speed of light in a vacuum, or 186,000 miles per second.

2. X-rays are usually referred to by their wavelength. The shorter the wavelength of an x-ray, the greater the penetrating power of that ray, or the "harder" it is said to be; and the longer the wavelength, the lesser the penetrating power or the "softer" the ray is said to be.

3. X-rays are produced by electrons bombarding a hard target.

4. X-rays cannot be reflected under normal conditions.

5. X-rays travel in straight lines. They are not deflected by electric or magnetic fields.

6. X-rays are absorbed by dense materials such as lead or steel, although the amount absorbed depends on the nature of the substance. It is this relative absorption that produces the shadows on the radiograph.

7. An x-ray beam is heterogeneous in nature, which means that it is composed of x-rays of different penetrating powers.

8. When certain materials are struck with x-rays, they give off visible light; this property is called fluorescence.

9. X-rays will ionize any gas they pass through.

10. X-rays and visible light both obey the law of inverse squares regarding their intensity at a particular distance from the source.

11. X-rays produce a variety of effects on the different kinds of tissue cells.

What is meant by wavelength and by wave frequency?

Wavelength is the distance between any point in one wave to the exact point in the next wave.

Wave frequency is the number of said wave crests passing any given point in one second.

If one can imagine in his own mind a specified distance between two points and if that distance is decreased, one can see that more of them would pass any given point in a given time interval. Thus the frequency would become greater because of the decrease in wavelength. Conversely, if the distance became longer, the frequency would become less because of the greater length of time to pass a given point in a given time interval.

What is meant by the electromagnetic spectrum?

Light, x-rays, and radiowaves are some of the energy waves of electric and magnetic influence. They are appropriately called electromagnetic waves and travel at a tremendous speed. All these forms of electromagnetic radiation are grouped according to their wavelengths in what is called the electromagnetic spectrum.

What is an x-ray tube?

An x-ray tube is a piece of apparatus specifically designed for the production of x-rays. It consists of the following: a thin wire filament (cathode), which when heated gives off free electrons; a metal target (anode), which is bombarded by the free electrons; a high-voltage supply, which propels the free electrons from cathode to anode with high velocity; and a glass tube with as complete a vacuum as possible to hold the anode and cathode.

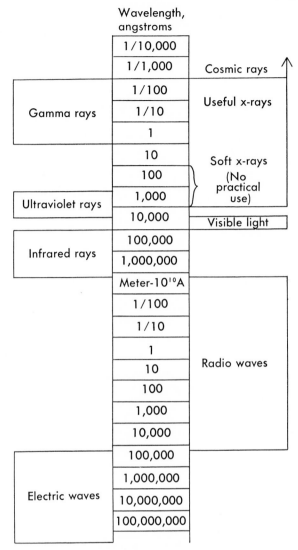

Fig. 10. Electromagnetic radiation.

How many electric circuits are there in an x-ray tube?

There are two electric circuits. The filament requires a low-voltage circuit to heat the filament wire and a high-voltage circuit to move the free electron across the vacuum to the anode.

What conditions are necessary for the production of x-rays?

There must be a source of free electrons. This is accomplished by heating the filament wire with low voltage and freeing electrons that are in orbit about the nucleus. To free the electrons the wire must glow. These free electrons are directed to a specific spot on the target by means of a focusing cup.

There must be a target to stop the flow

of electrons. The target must be of material that resists melting under the high heat produced when the electrons strike the target.

There must be a high-voltage supply to propel the free electrons from the filament to the target. This is accomplished by making the cathode a high negative charge. This negative charge will repel the electrons and drive them across the tube. The positive charge attracts the negative electrons.

There must be a high vacuum. A vacuum will prevent a charge in space and oxidation of the filament.

What is meant by hard and soft x-rays?

Hard x-rays are those that have a short wavelength and great frequency. They are produced by high kilovoltage and are more penetrating.

Soft x-rays are those that have a long wavelength and lesser frequency. These are produced by low kilovoltage and are more easily absorbed.

How are x-rays produced?

A stream of rapidly moving, negatively charged electrons strike a positively charged target. While it has been stated that the bombardment of this target results in the production of x-rays, we believe it more nearly correct to say that the deceleration (or abrupt stoppage) of these electrons produces x-rays. The amount of this electron steam that is converted into heat is 99.9 percent. The remainder, 0.1 percent, is converted into x-rays.

How can the technologist control the production of x-rays?

X-ray production can be controlled by mastering the two electric circuits in the x-ray tube. The wavelength of the x-rays are controlled by the high-voltage circuit. If the applied high voltage across the tube is reduced, the wavelength becomes longer. By controlling the output of free electrons from the filament, the current flow across the tube can be varied.

Why are x-rays called heterogeneous?

All x-ray beams that exit from the x-ray tube do not have the same wavelength or frequency. Because of this phenomenon of the x-ray beam being made up of different wavelengths, the x-ray beam is considered to be heterogeneous.

What is meant by the quality of the x-ray beam?

The quality of the x-ray beam is its penetrating power. The penetrating power is dependent upon the voltage applied across the tube.

What is the law of conservation of energy?

The law of conservation of energy states that energy can neither be created nor destroyed but can be changed from one form to another, for example, water into steam.

It has been stated that with all the energy in the world the total amount never changes. If this is true, with what sources of energy do we contend?

The sources of energy are heat, light, electric, mechanical, chemical, molecular, atomic, and nuclear. All these may change from one form to another but never lose any of the total energy.

In the diagrammatic drawings in Fig. 11 are signs used in electric circuitry. Can you identify them?

Electrons usually flow freely in the electric circuit. Their progress is either helped or retarded by the resistance. What materials would you suggest to assist or resist the flow of electricity?

Most metals are considered to be good conductors of electricity. Copper is the one with which we are most experienced.

Materials that resist the flow of electricity are plastic, wood, glass, and rubber.

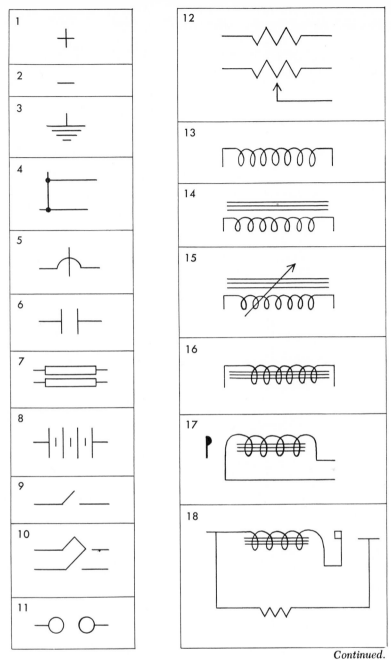

Continued.

Fig. 11. Diagrammatic representation of terms common to electric circuitry. The corresponding literal terms are as follows:

1. Positive charge
2. Negative charge
3. Grounding
4. Connected wires
5. Crossed wires (electrically not connected)
6. Condenser
7. Fuses
8. Battery
9. Single switch
10. Two-pole switch

11. Sphere gap
12. Fixed resistance (above) and variable resistance (below)
13. Fixed induction coil
14. Induction coil with iron core
15. Variable induction coil
16. Choke coil
17. Relay
18. Stabilizer with resistance coil in shunt

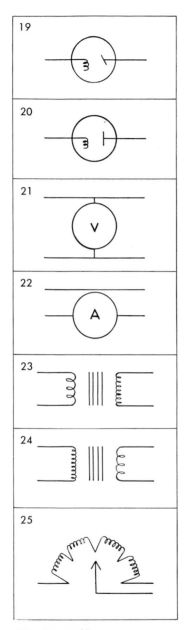

Fig. 11, cont'd.

19. X-ray tube
20. Valve tube
21. Volt meter (across the circuit)
22. Ampere meter (in circuit)
23. Step-up transformer
24. Step-down transformer
25. Rheostat (ampere selector)

26. Autotransformer
27. Circuit breaker
28. Rheostat
29. Foot switch
30. Selenium cell
31. Push button contact
32. Contactor

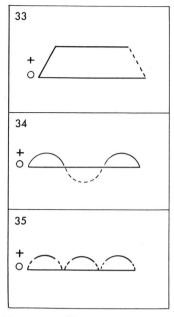
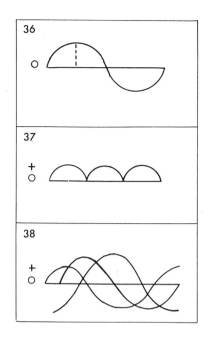

Fig. 11, cont'd.
33. Direct current (DC)
34. Half-wave current (rectified)
35. Full-wave current (mechanically rectified)
36. Alternating current (AC)
37. Full-wave current (rectified)
38. Three-phase current

These are called nonconductors, insulators, or dielectrics.

What is meant by characteristic radiation?

Radiation may be produced by bombarding metal targets with high-speed electrons. The deceleration of these electrons by the targets produces radiation of various wavelengths. It has been found that certain metals will emit a wavelength particular to that metal. This is called characteristic radiation and refers to the wavelength characteristic of that particular metal target.

What are roentgen, rad, and MPD?

The roentgen is an international unit of radiation exposure and is often referred to as the *r* dose. The quantity of radiation is such that the associated corpuscular emission in 0.001293 gram of air produces, in air, ions carrying an electrostatic unit quantity of electricity of either sign.

The rad is a unit of absorbed dose and is 100 ergs per gram.

Maximum permissible dose (MPD) for an individual is the largest dose accumulated that, in light of present knowledge, carries a negligible probability of severe somatic or genetic injuries. Persons working with radiation may compute their MPD by using the formula 5(N-18) rads, where N equals the age of the worker. Thus, if a technician were 22 years of age, we could substitute 5(22-18) rads, or 20 rads, as the MPD of the worker.

What is dose rate, and how may it be controlled?

Dose rate for practical purposes may be considered as the amount of radiation given to a patient over a period of time. It is the rate (r per minute) times the length of exposure. It may be controlled by four factors—kilovoltage, milliamperage, amount and type of filtration, and target-skin distance.

Define primary radiation.

Primary radiation is considered to be that radiation emitted directly from the target. It is caused by the deceleration of the high-speed electrons by the target. It consists of x-ray wavelengths of different intensities and has its characteristic wavelength of the metal.

What is meant by secondary and scattered radiation?

When an x-ray beam strikes an object and penetrates it, the beam changes in wavelength in passing through the object because of the partial absorption of the beam. The emergent beam from the object is called secondary radiation.

Scattered radiation is understood to be the change of direction of the radiation from its original course after striking an object.

What is remnant radiation?

Remnant radiation has been defined as the radiation that emerges from the radiated object and reaches the film. This occurs after the partial absorption of the primary ray (secondary radiation) and the primary radiation, which penetrates and is never changed.

What is absorbed radiation?

As the primary radiation strikes an object and penetrates it, some of the initial force, or intensity, is decreased. The resultant emergent wavelength is longer. The change in wavelength intensity between the primary and secondary radiation is caused by the absorption of energy by the struck part. In some instances the wavelength may be of such length that the part may completely absorb it.

What is meant by unmodified scattering?

A single x-ray photon entering an object could strike an atom of this matter but not dislodge it from its orbit. The orbital electron remains in its shell either because of the glancing blow from the x-ray photon or because it is firmly held in place. However, the x-ray photon does change its direction of flight as a result of the glancing blow. This is called unmodified scattering. The x-ray photon does not lose any of its energy when striking the orbital electron.

What is meant by the Compton effect?

Compton effect occurs when a photon enters an atomic structure and collides with an electron orbiting in an outer shell with such force as to dislodge the electron. The photon then proceeds in a different direction from the one in which it entered. In striking the electron, a certain amount of the photon energy is transferred to the electron so that, when the photon emerges in a changed direction, the energy has been decreased and the wavelength lengthened.

What is photoelectric effect?

Photoelectric effect is a reaction that occurs when an incident low-energy photon interacts with an inner-orbital electron, driving it out of the energy shell. The entire energy of the incident photon is given to the electron and the incident photon ceases to exist.

What is Bremsstrahlung radiation?

Bremsstrahlung radiation occurs when an electron passes near the positively charged nucleus of an atom and its velocity decreases because of the attraction of the electron and nucleus. This results in a loss of energy expressed as Bremsstrahlung.

How can x-rays be detected?

X-rays can be detected in many ways:
1. *Photographically.* X-rays affect the

emulsion on the film and can be seen when the film is developed.

2. *By fluorescence.* X-rays have the ability to cause certain chemicals to glow when in the presence of x-rays.

3. *By ionization.* X-rays have the property of ionizing gases.

4. *Physiologically.* X-rays will cause skin to redden (as in a sunburn). They can destroy tissues.

5. *Chemically.* X-rays have the ability to change the color of certain chemicals when the chemicals are struck with x-rays over a certain time interval.

What is meant by a hot filament tube?

A hot filament tube is a thermionic vacuum tube that provides a heated filament wire furnishing a source of free electrons. The filament is heated by a predetermined filament current; thus, the electron cloud is controlled.

What are the electric factors under which the x-ray filament operates?

The filament of the x-ray tube usually operates at approximately 10 volts and 3 to 5 amperes.

What can be said about the life of the filament wire?

The life of the filament wire will vary with its use. As the tube is constantly used, the evaporation of the wire metal causes it to become thinner. The thinner the wire, the greater the resistance produced in the wire. Many technologists inadvertently leave the x-ray machine in the "on position." Although the filament may be at low voltage and will come to full electron flow only when the rotor switch is pressed, it should be understood that the low heat also causes evaporation of the filament wire.

What types of anodes are in use today?

There are two types of anodes in use today, stationary and rotating.

The stationary anode is composed of a piece of copper into which a piece of tungsten metal has been embedded. The anode is placed so that the target is directly across from, and aligned with, the focused filament wire. Copper is used as the base because of its high heat-conducting characteristic, whereas tungsten is used for the production of x-rays because of its high melting point and high atomic number.

The rotating anode is constructed of a beveled tungsten disk attached to an induction motor shaft. The beveled edge of the disk is again, like the stationary anode, aligned with the focused cathode filament. During the exposure the target rotates to present a new section to the beam of electrons. The energy of the x-ray beam is then distributed over the entire face of the target.

What is meant by a double-focus tube?

A double-focus tube is that in which two focal spots are utilized. These are called the small and large focal spots. The focal spots are controlled by the length of the focused filament wire (usually two).

What effect does the kilovoltage have on the flow of electrons in the x-ray tube?

The freeing of electrons from the heated filament wire depends upon the voltage and amperage applied. For any given setting, a specific heat is maintained and a specific cloud of electrons freed. If kilovoltage is applied to this filament, the electrons are propelled across the tube. Low kilovoltage propels only a certain percentage of free electrons across the tube. As the kilovoltage is increased, more and more electrons are accelerated across the target until the kilovoltage propels all the electrons as they are emitted from the wire. When this phase is reached, the condition is known as producing a saturation current.

Are there disadvantages to using a rotating anode tube?

Yes. There are some disadvantages, but the advantages certainly compensate for them. The disadvantages are as follows:

1. Since the rotating mechanism is inside the tube envelope, there is a need for a complicated system to produce electric induction for rotation of the target.
2. Certainly the manufacture and purchase of a rotating anode tube is more expensive than a stationary anode.
3. Since the target area of the rotating anode is larger, the heating area is larger and the tube cooling is longer.
4. There can be no instantaneous exposure using rotating anode tubes. There is a certain period of time delay while the target reaches its operating speed. This is overcome by the use of a double-switch exposure handle, in which one switch controls the speed of the rotor and the other the exposure.

What are the actual focal spot and the effective focal spot?

The actual focal spot is the area that is bombarded by the high-speed electron stream and, when projected in its arc of declination, is approximately three times longer than its width.

The effective focal spot is the spot that is measured directly below the target area bombarded by the high-speed electrons and at right angles to the stream of electrons.

How can one determine the size of the focal spot in the x-ray tube?

A pinhole camera could be used to determine the size of the focal spot. This is accomplished by placing a sheet of lead with a perfect pinhole in it directly under the tube target an equidistance from the target and film. An exposure of low kilo-voltage and milliamperage is made. The film is processed, and the actual effective focal spot can be measured. One must remember in measuring the focal spot to subtract two times the diameter of the pinhole from the size of the spot. As a rule, however, the operator may depend upon the tube manufacturer to supply the focal spot size.

In radiography one often hears about, and is instructed in, the use of focal spots for radiographic exposures. Why are they important?

The use of the correct focal spot has two factors to consider. In the geometry of image formation we learn that the smaller the focal spot, the sharper the radiographic detail; the smaller the focal spot, the less penumbra is seen. Second, the choice of focal spots will, in some measure, determine the exposure to be made. The exposure must take into consideration the tube rating and capacity.

What is a tube-rating chart?

A tube-rating chart is a chart provided by the manufacturer for operation of that particular x-ray tube. The chart is based on a particular tube, specific focal spots, and type of rectification. It is used to determine the limits of safe operation of the tube for any exposure using time, milliamperage, and kilovoltage. Usually in the chart the horizontal base line represents the unit of time, the vertical line the range of kilovoltage, and the angled lines the milliamperage. To find the same exposure rate the technologist determines the kvp to be used on the vertical line and follows it across the chart to the desired milliamperage and down to the time of maximum exposure.

Suppose that an exposure using 65 kvp and 300 ma was to be made. The technologist wishes to change factors to 85 kvp and use 300 ma because of the patient's con-

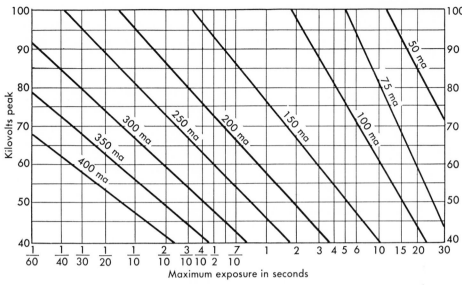

Fig. 12. Tube-rating chart for a 4.5 mm. focal spot on a full-wave generator.

dition. What is the maximum exposure time to be used?

If we draw a line across the diagram from 65 kvp to the bisecting point of 300-ma line, we will find that the exposure time is slightly longer than one-tenth second. For radiographic purposes, unless we were to use an impulse timer, one-tenth second would be the maximum time for that exposure. However, by raising the kvp we will repeat the procedure and find that the line drawn from 85 kvp will cross the 300-ma line at one-fortieth second. This is the maximum exposure time for this technique.

With the same diagram, can an exposure using 65 kvp, 300 ma, and one-fifth second be changed to use 75 kvp at 300 ma?

No. If the rule of thumb is utilized for exposure, we know that when the exposure is increased by 10 kvp the time of exposure may be halved. If a line is drawn from 75 kvp across to the 300-ma line, it can be seen that the maximum time of exposure is less than one-twentieth sec-

ond. Hence, another set of exposure factors must be determined.

We have considered the fact that 99 percent of the energy is converted at the target because of the deceleration of the high-speed electrons. What is meant by "heat units to the tube"? How are they produced?

Heat units are a measure of the total amount of heat generated within the x-ray tube for any given exposure or series of exposures. The heat storage capacity of the x-ray tube is computed by the tube manufacturer and shown in the thermal characteristic chart of the tube. Heat units are determined in units representing the product of the kilovoltage times the milliamperage times the time in seconds for single-phase generators. For three-phase generators this product must be multiplied by 1.35 to attain the heat units applicable.

Both x-ray and valve tubes are thermionic diode tubes capable of producing x-rays. Explain the difference between construc-

tion of the modern valve tube and the x-ray tube.

In the early days of valve tube manufacture the construction of the tube was similar to that of the x-ray tube in that it utilized the in-line process of cathode and anode. Today this valve tube is obsolete. The modern valve tube is constructed so that the filament consists of a longer and larger coil of wire and is placed in a longitudinal plane. Around this filament wire is the anode in the shape of a cylinder, thus enabling all the electrons emitted from the filament to be drawn to the anode. The valve tube operates as a low resistance to the voltage flow because of the large amounts of filament emission.

Therefore, if the resistance is low, there will be a low-voltage drop across the tube (in comparison to the high-voltage drop in the x-ray tube) for any given current.

With all the care in tube manufacture, why do x-ray tubes fail?

X-ray tubes usually fail because of human errors. Although it is true that there may be some manufacturing defects, the answer generally lies a little closer to the operation of the equipment. The majority of x-ray tubes fail because the filament burns out. This is caused by the overloading of the filament circuit or the continuous heating of the filament wire during normal usage. Again, one must be cautioned about the problem of leaving the x-ray machine turned on. Although the filament is at low voltage, there is a certain amount of burning off, or evaporation, of the metal.

The tube may fail because of excessive heat units being applied to the tube. The condition exists when serial radiography is being accomplished. Excessive heat units to the anode could cause it to glow and emit electrons. In the self-rectified unit the inverse voltage phase would then flow from anode to cathode.

Overloading, to some degree, results in damage to the target. The impact of the high-speed electrons causes tiny depressions on the face of the tube. This is called pitting and results in x-rays of uneven wavelengths being emitted from the tube.

Failure of the rotor and failure of the target to reach maximum rotor speed before the exposure is made result in target pitting and complete breakdown of the target itself.

With the advent of high kvp (125 to 150), the danger of damage to other metal parts of the x-ray tube exists. This destruction causes vaporization of the part and a deposit of a metallic coating inside the tube. The pressure of this metallic coating can produce a puncture of the glass envelope.

What is meant by heat dissipation rate?

Heat dissipation rate is the cooling characteristics or ability of the x-ray tube to cool. It is determined by the manufacturer for that particular tube under normal operating conditions.

How are x-ray tubes cooled?

In the manufacture of x-ray tubes the anode and cathode are encased in a glass vacuum envelope and immersed in oil. The heat from the tube is conducted by the oil to the metal housing. The small fan circulates the room air over the tube housing and improves the conduction of heat through the air.

High-voltage therapy tubes are cooled by pumping oil into the anode and around the tube. The oil is then recirculated through a cooling unit, which reduces the heat of the oil. The oil is then pumped again through the anode and tube.

What do you consider half-value layer to be?

Half-value layer is the thickness of any given material that will reduce the primary radiation to one half its intensity. This is one method of determining the quality of the radiation beam.

List all the component parts of the full-wave, four-valve rectified x-ray circuit in Fig. 13. For what is the spinning top used?

The spinning top is a flat circular piece of metal that is mounted on a pivot and has a small hole near the edge. The top is placed on an x-ray film and rotated at a normal spin. A predetermined exposure time (usually one-tenth second) is made. The film is processed, and the dots are counted. With an exposure time of one-tenth second and a 60-cycle current (120 impulses) in operation, you should have

twelve dots if the machine is full-wave rectified. There will be six dots if a self-rectified unit is used. This procedure can be used to test the operation of the valve tubes and/or the efficiency of the x-ray timer.

What is electrostatics?

Electrostatics is the branch of physics that concerns electric charges that are stationary or resting.

Most fields of science have causes and effects. The field of electrostatics has its causes and effects that produce laws that govern the science. What are they?

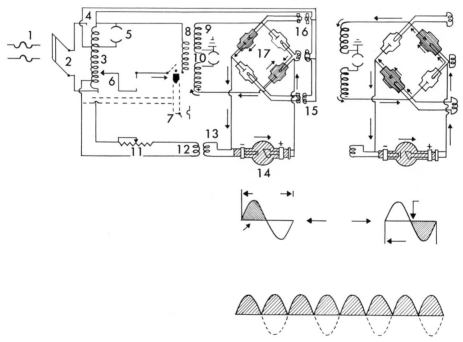

Fig. 13. A full-wave four-valve rectified x-ray circuit with first and second half-cycles. The component parts are as follows:

1. Fuses
2. Line switch
3. Auto transformer
4. Line voltage compensator
5. Voltage compensator meter
6. X-ray voltage control
7. X-ray switch
8. X-ray transformer, primary
9. X-ray transformer, secondary
10. Grounded milliammeter
11. X-ray filament resistor (ma control)
12. X-ray filament transformer, primary
13. X-ray filament transformer, secondary
14. X-ray tube
15. Filament transformer, primary
16. Filament transformer, secondary
17. Valve tubes

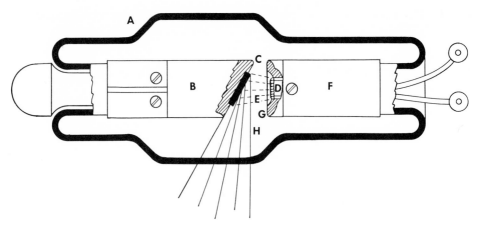

Fig. 14. Stationary anode x-ray tube. Names of important parts follow:

A. Glass envelope
B. Anode
C. Tungsten target
D. Filament of x-ray tube

E. Electron stream
F. Cathode
G. Focusing cup
H. Primary radiation (x-ray)

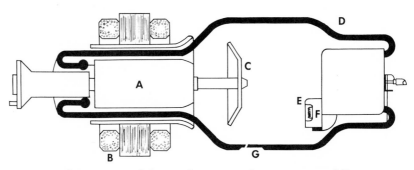

Fig. 15. Rotating anode x-ray tube. Names of important parts follow:

A. Rotor
B. Stator windings
C. Tungsten disk anode
D. Glass window

E. Focusing cup
F. Filament
G. X-ray window

The first law of electrostatics that we may consider is akin to that of magnetism; that is, like charges repel each other while unlike charges attract.

Electric charges exist only on the outside of the conductors. They tend to concentrate on a curved surface at a point where the curve is the greatest.

Only negative charges can move in a solid conductor.

What factors would you expect to find in making up an electric circuit?

The factors that make up an electric circuit are three in number:

1. There must be a difference in potential between two points in the circuit. This means that there is an abundance of electrons at one end and a deficit at the other end.
2. There must be a certain amount of

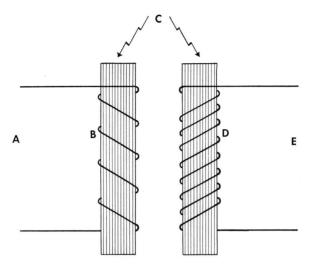

Fig. 16. Open core transformer. Because of the greater number of turns of wire in the secondary side in relation to those of the primary side, this is a step-up transformer. Names of transformer parts follow:

A. Incoming line to primary side
B. Primary side of transformer
C. Soft iron cores with no visible connections

D. Secondary side of transformer
E. Load voltage

current flowing through the conductor. In the case of a battery-operated circuit, the current flows in one direction only and is strong when first put into operation. However, as the time of operation increases, the strength of the current decreases.

3. With any material there is a characteristic resistance. Materials will vary in their resistance, some having a high resistance and others having a low resistance.

Label the important parts in Fig. 14 (stationary anode) and Fig. 15 (rotating anode tubes).

Identify the type of transformer and label the parts in Figs. 16 to 18.

Transformers are made to operate as efficiently as possible. Still there are energy losses in the operation of them. Can you name the types of transformer losses?

Losses from transformer material result

in the loss of energy because of resistance in the coil of wire. The smaller the wire, the higher the resistance.

When currents are induced into the coil of wire, the coil gets hot. This heat removes electric energy from the current in the transformer coils. This phenomenon is called eddy current loss.

Transformers operate on alternating current and in working constantly change the magnetic field of force while also changing the polarity of the field. The constant change in the transformer causes heat in the core. The heat in the core causes a loss in efficiency of the transformer. This is called hysteresis loss.

A series of x-rays using the same technique are taken, and the resultant films show densities of varying darkness. You believe the timer to be inaccurate. What methods can be employed to determine the correctness of the time?

The technologist may use the spinning top or a stopwatch to test the accuracy of

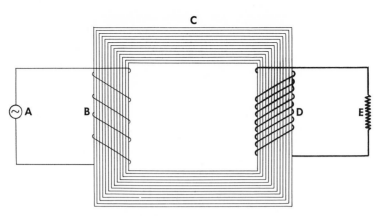

Fig. 17. Closed core transformer. Names of transformer parts follow:

A. Incoming line to primary side
B. Primary side of transformer
C. Closed core of laminated metal plates

D. Secondary side of transformer
E. Load voltage

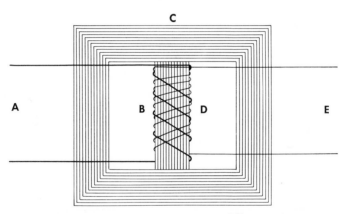

Fig. 18. Shell type transformer. Names of transformer parts follow:

A. Incoming line to primary side
B. Primary side of transformer
C. Shell type core with center post (The core is constructed of laminated steel with both

the primary and secondary coils wound around the center post.)
D. Secondary side of transformer
E. Load voltage

the timer. A service man may use a cycle counter in addition to using the previous method.

What method is used to stabilize the incoming line voltage to the x-ray machine?

The line voltage compensator is used to correct the fluctuations of the incoming line. By adjusting the number of turns on the primary side of the transformer, the line voltage can be made to read correctly.

Transformers are classified as step-up or step-down transformers. Can you name the various transformers in the x-ray electric circuit and classify them?

The filament transformers to the x-ray and valve tube filaments are step-down transformers. The high-tension transformer is a step-up transformer. The autotransformer may be either a step-up or step-down transformer, depending upon how the kvp is being varied. The incoming line pole transformer might also be included as a step-down transformer.

Why are fuses placed in the electric circuit?

Fuses are placed in the electric circuit to prevent damage to the x-ray machine as a result of an overload or shortage within the circuit. If an overload occurs and the amperage increases, the resultant heat will melt the wire within the fuse.

Is a circuit breaker the same as a fuse?

Yes. Essentially, the circuit breaker is placed in the circuit to prevent damage to the x-ray machine from overloaded and short circuits. However, the circuit breaker may be reset manually if tripped and thus restore the circuit to normal use, whereas the fuse must be replaced when burned out.

What types of current are found in electricity?

There are two types of current used in electricity, direct current (DC), which only flows in one direction, and alternating current (AC), which changes its flow of direction at specified intervals.

Can transformers work on direct current?

No. Transformers work on alternating current. If direct current is the only kind available, an interrupter or converter must be used to change the direct current.

We speak of transformers being step-up or step-down transformers. What is the difference?

In general, the difference between these transformers lies in their construction. The step-up transformer is constructed with more turns of wire in the secondary coil than in the primary. The step-down transformer is made just the opposite, having more turns of wire in the primary than in the secondary coil.

What is pulsating direct current?

Pulsating direct current flows in the x-ray circuit from the valve tube to the x-ray tube. It is called pulsating direct current because the negative half of the cycle has been rectified to a positive flow of current. Since the alternating current builds up and recedes, the current is never at the same current strength.

What is meant by transformer ratio?

Transformer ratio is the relation of the number of turns of the primary coil of wire to the number of turns on the secondary coil of wire.

What is a sphere gap?

A sphere gap is an instrument that is placed in the high-tension circuit to measure the voltage in the high-tension circuit.

What is a ballistic meter?

A ballistic meter is a device installed in modern x-ray equipment to register the product of the milliamperage times the time. In other words, it denotes the milliampere-seconds or actual current flowing through the tube. The ballistic meter is only used during periods of short exposure. The meter, because it is so sensitive, must be used with an impulse timer or an electronic timer.

List the component parts of the circuit in Fig. 19.

What is a linear accelerator?

Linear acceleration is a way of accelerating charged partcles to high energies by having the particles receive a succession of small energy increments. The simple linear accelerator consists of an ion source and a series of hollow metallic cylinders or drift tubes of gradually increasing lengths. Alternate tubes of positive and negative charge are connected together, and the two sets of tubes are in

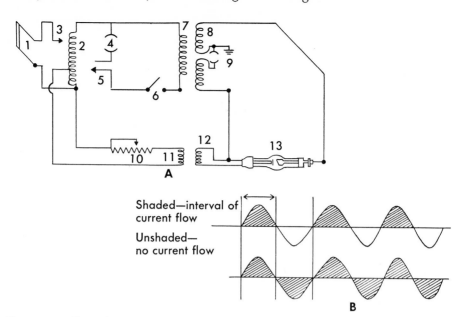

Fig. 19. A self-rectified circuit. A, Diagram of the circuit. B, Voltage across an x-ray tube. Correct identifications follow:

1. Line switch
2. Auto transformer
3. Line voltage compensator
4. Voltage compensator meter
5. X-ray voltage control
6. X-ray switch (timer)
7. X-ray transformer, primary

8. X-ray transformer, secondary
9. Grounded milliammeter
10. X-ray filament resistor (ma control)
11. X-ray filament transformer, primary
12. X-ray filament transformer, secondary
13. X-ray tube

turn connected to a high-frequency oscillator producing a certain wavelength.

If a positively charged particle such as a proton is used at the beginning of the accelerator and the first tube is negatively charged, the particle accelerates as it passes through the space between the tubes and gains energy corresponding to the potential difference between the two tubes. While the proton is inside the second tube it does not accelerate but retains the same velocity and energy because the proton is in a region of uniform field. This is the reason that the cylinders are called "drift tubes." The drift tube is constructed such that during the time it takes the proton to "drift" through it, the potential changes from negative to positive. As the proton emerges, cylinder two quickly

changes to positive and cylinder three to negative; thus the proton accelerates again. This process repeats itself throughout the length of the accelerator. The final energy of the proton after passing through the tubes is equal to the sum of the energy increments gained at the spacing between each tube. Since the oscillator frequency remains constant and the velocity of the proton increases as it progresses through the accelerators, it is necessary to make each successive tube longer. This allows the proton and wavelength arriving at each tube exit to be in unison.

Linear accelerators are used for medical purposes to accelerate electrons that can be used for both radiation therapy and isotope production.

16 RADIATION PROTECTION

Since shortly after the discovery of x-rays it has been known that excessive radiation exposure would cause tissue damage. Over the years numerous tests and experiments have been performed for the purpose of gathering information relative to the hazards of radiation. Much has been learned and published for the benefit of those dealing with radiation. In today's society, with the testing of atomic weapons and the increasing usage of radiation in the medical field and industry, even more information is being correlated. To those of us within the profession, it is of vital importance to know the hazards encountered and the best methods of reducing the dangers to the patients and ourselves.

Radiation causes two general kinds of effects on humans. What are they?

General radiation effects are somatic and genetic. Somatic is injury to the body tissues from radiation, and genetic is damage to the reproductive organs, damage not readily apparent but becoming evident in future generations as hereditary defects.

How are the ionizing radiation and radiation exposure to mankind categorized?

1. Natural radiation, two external sources—cosmic radiation and gamma radiation from materials naturally present in the earth and naturally occurring radionuclides deposited within the body
2. Radiation from medical procedures
3. Radiation applied in research on human subjects
4. Occupational irradiation
5. Manmade environmental radiation

Radiation exposure has a particular meaning as opposed to absorbed dose. Define each.

Exposure is a measure of the quantity of radiation at a given point based upon its ability to ionize air. Absorbed dose is the energy absorbed from the radiation per unit mass of the material in question.

To what does maximum permissible dose refer?

Maximum permissible dose (MPD) refers to the amount of radiation absorbed by the body in a stated period of time without causing appreciable body injury. This is for radiation to the total body area, not a' confined area, since a smaller area can tolerate more radiation than the overall body, with the exception of the gonadal area.

For general irradiation of the whole body, which are the "critical organs"?

1. Blood-forming organs (red bone marrow)

2. Lens of the eye
3. Gonads

If external irradiation of restricted parts of the body is done, then the skin becomes an additional critical organ.

How is exposure dose stated?

Exposure to x-, beta, or gamma radiation is stated in rads. The total depends on the quantity of radiation and the type of radiation used. For all purposes the radiation from x, beta, or gamma sources are given the same value.

What is the purpose and goal of the National Committee on Radiation Protection and Measurement?

The purpose is to study the effects of radiation and to develop recommendations from these studies for the populace to keep the exposures from radiation well below a level at which adverse effects are likely.

In the manufacture of x-ray tubes, the housing has a safe limit. What constitutes this safe limit?

All enclosures, or tube housings, must be constructed so that the leakage of radiation at a distance of 1 meter from the target cannot exceed 100 mr in an hour when the tube is operated at any of its specified ratings.

Define half-value layer.

Half-value layer is the thickness of any material necessary to reduce a given amount of intensity to one half. Any material will reduce radiation, but the amount of material in a half-value layer will depend upon its ability to absorb radiation.

Define exposure dose rate.

Exposure dose rate is the amount of time necessary to receive a given amount of radiation; it is dependent upon the source and type of radiation being utilized. X-, beta, and gamma radiation has been given a quality factor of 1, whereas a neutron source has a factor of 10 and alpha particles a quality factor of 2. This means that in a given amount of time exposure to neutrons will cause an exposure dose ten times greater than exposure to x-rays in the same amount of time.

What is the maximum amount of radiation leakages allowed for therapeutic tube housings?

The radiation leakage at a distance of 1 meter from the target cannot exceed 1 r in one hour. At a distance of 5 cm. from any point on the surface of the housing accessible to the patient it cannot exceed 30 r in one hour when the tube is operated at any of its specified ratings.

Name and define the units of measurement used in dealing with radiation.

Roentgen (r). That quantity of x-rays or gamma rays in which each corpuscular emission per 0.001293 gram of air produces in air ions carrying one electrostatic unit of electricity of either sign.

Rad (radiation absorbed dose). The measure of the amount of energy imparted to matter by any ionizing radiation per unit mass of irradiated material at the place of interest; 1 rad is equal to 100 ergs of absorbed energy per gram of absorbing material.

RBE (relative biologic effectiveness). Term used to show that different types of radiation affect biologic systems differently. It compares the effects of x-rays or gamma rays to the effects of any other radiation.

Rem (roentgen equivalent, man). Unit of human biologic dose as a result of exposure to one or more types of ionizing radiation. Dose in rem is equal to dose in rad × RBE.

Curie. Unit of radioactivity in which the number of disintegrations per second is 3.7×10^{10}.

What are the three most practical methods of radiation protection to be observed by persons working with ionizing radiation?

By remembering proper time, distance, and shielding the radiation worker can keep his exposure to radiation at low levels.

What are the methods of radiation monitoring?

Pocket dosimeters and film badges are the two most prominent means of radiation monitoring. Pocket dosimeters are more accurate but do not allow permanent records to be kept. Film badges are worn by the personnel and periodically (dependent upon the amount of work performed in the department) are checked against a film exposed to a known amount of radiation in a densitometer. This permits permanent records to be kept.

Where does the largest amount of radiation (scattered) usually originate during fluoroscopy?

Scattered radiation during fluoroscopy usually originates in the patient. As the radiation strikes the tabletop and the patient, it glances off in all directions.

Whenever it is known or suspected that a person has received exposure in excess of the maximum permissible dose, what procedure should be followed?

In any case in which it is suspected that a person has been excessively exposed, a blood count should be done immediately to prepare for the detection of any resultant changes at a later date. Records should be kept of reports of physical examinations and blood counts.

During diagnostic radiology the radiation is absorbed in the tissues by which process?

Photoelectric absorption. This is the process in which all the energy of the incident photon is used up in dislodging the electron from its shell, giving it kinetic energy.

Photoelectric absorption results in true absorption of the incident photon.

There has been established a maximum permissible dose, but is there a minimum dose level?

No known levels have been established as a minimum dose, below which radiation will have no effect. Any level, or grade, of radiation will cause some effect because of its ability to be absorbed by body tissues. It is known that absorbed dosage in excess of 25 rads to the whole body in one exposure will produce a discernible, temporary depression of the manufacture of white blood cells.

What are the maximum permissible dose rates for occupational personnel?

The maximum permissible dose for whole-body irradiation from all occupational sources is 5 rems in one year, or 100 millirads per week. For the skin it shall not exceed 0.5 rem; for the hands, 75 rems. Occupational exposures for pregnant women shall not exceed 0.5 rem to the fetus for the entire gestation period.

What are some rules governing radiation exposure to the patient during fluoroscopy?

When using conventional fluoroscopy, dark adaptation is of paramount importance since incorrect adaptation will necessitate undue exposure to the patient. All tabletops should be no less than 15 inches from the tube, and the dose rate to the patient should be less than 10 r per minute. A fluoroscopic tube and a restricted field size are necessary.

When does a radiation hazard exist?

Any situation in which persons might receive radiation in excess of the maximum permissible dose is likely to be a hazard.

Why is it important that persons from 17 to 30 years of age be protected as much as possible from excessive amounts of radiation?

It is believed that during these years the average person will deliver children into the world. Excessive dosages of radiation will damage the chromosomes of the reproductive cells, and the hereditary material will be transmitted from parent to offspring by the genes that are contained in the chromosomes.

What are the maximum permissible dosages allowed for nonoccupational personnel?

The maximum permissible dosages allowed are one tenth of those of occupational personnel, or 0.25 mr per hour or 0.5 rem per year.

What is a primary rule to be followed when dealing with machines that produce ionizing radiation?

A basic and important rule to be followed is that no device or machine producing radiation should ever be used by persons who are unfamiliar with the operation and the radiation safety precautions to be followed.

Why do we use filtration in radiography? What is added filtration?

Filtration is useful in radiography because it filters or absorbs the long, soft wavelengths that otherwise would be absorbed by the tissues. Added filtration is any material added to the tube port to attenuate the beam. The usual added filter material is aluminum and is normally 2.5 mm. An increase from 1 mm. to 3 mm. of aluminum will reduce the exposure rate to the patient by approximately one fourth. The addition of aluminum causes only a slight loss in radiographic density and contrast.

Certain materials have been designated as those to be used for protection when working with diagnostic radiation. What are they?

In most instances the radiologist and the technologist are required to wear lead rubber aprons and gloves, each having an equivalent protection value equal to 0.25 mm. lead. Lead, being one of the best absorbers of radiation, is mixed with rubber to afford a lightweight protective device for personnel and patients.

What are the two types of filters used in diagnostic radiology?

The two types of filters used are the inherent and the added filters. Inherent filtration is that which is afforded by the window of the x-ray tube and any permanent tube enclosure. Added filtration is that which is placed in addition to the inherent, usually made of aluminum.

In the process of radiographing patients, radiation of a characteristic nature is created or given off. What happens to this characteristic radiation?

As the photon strikes the tissues it creates radiation characteristics of the tissue, and these radiation characteristics are totally absorbed in the tissue.

It has been stated that the absorption of radiation from diagnostic machines is by photoelectric effect. Is this true for exposure to radiation therapy?

No. The process of absorption by radiation therapy is Compton absorption process. There is a difference because of the nature of the beam and the reaction of tissue to this change.

During fluoroscopy, where is the safest position for the fluoroscopist and technician?

The fluoroscopist should be utilizing a small field size and lead rubber shields, and thus the safest place would be over the fluoroscopic screen. This screen has a small amount of protection, and utilizing a small field should be safe. The technician should be in the control booth or, if required to be in the room, should wear a lead apron and should stand behind the radiologist or far enough away from the source to take advantage of the inverse square law.

Which type of fluoroscopic tube arrangement results in the least amount of scatter radiation being absorbed by the fluoroscopist?

When the fluoroscopic tube is mounted above the tabletop and is pointed at an image intensifier beneath the tabletop, scatter that originated from the patient's skin surface will directly expose the operator standing beside the patient. When the fluoroscopic tube is mounted beneath the table, however, much of the scattered radiation from the patient is absorbed by the patient, resulting in less exposure to the operator.

When performing "test exposures" for a portable x-ray examination, what is the safest procedure to follow in order to minimize the absorption of scatter radiation to yourself and patient?

To eliminate the possibility of unnecessarily radiating yourself or the patient during the "test exposures," the following steps should be taken:

1. Wear lead apron.
2. Close collimator completely.
3. If window is nearby, aim tube out of window to allow any radiation not absorbed by collimator to escape without obstruction.
4. If no window is present, place folded lead apron over closed collimator to absorb any radiation that may escape and aim tube away from personnel.

What is the most dangerous time for radiation exposure to the unborn fetus?

It is during the first trimester (first three months) that the fetus is most susceptible to somatic injury, and it is therefore during this time that no x-ray procedure, except in case of emergency, should be performed on the mother.

17 RADIATION THERAPY

Soon after the utilization of x-rays for diagnostic purposes began, observers noted a side effect that was to lead to the eventual use of the x-ray in the treatment of disease. The long radiation exposures necessary to produce images on the plates were the apparent cause of skin lesions suffered by patients and operators who were exposed to rays from the unshielded tubes. By testing radiation doses and exploring the effects on a variety of chronic skin diseases, researchers discovered that certain skin lesions responded favorably to the beam, and they consequently began to explore the possible therapeutic advantages of the x-ray.

The properties of ionization by the x-ray produce certain biologic changes in living tissue. Excessive amounts of radiation inflict indiscriminate damage on tissues that is especially marked during cell reproduction. However, by controlling the amount of radiation, it is possible to limit radiation's damaging effect to certain cells. Since tumor cells reproduce more rapidly than normal cells, their susceptibility to the ionizing rays is also increased; these tissue cells are said to be "radiosensitive," easily destroyed at levels of radiation that will not seriously harm normal cells. Radiation therapy is most successful where risk to healthy tissue is negligible, such as in treating localized tumors in an accessible position in the body.

Why are x-rays useful in the treatment of disease?

X-rays are useful because they can penetrate tissue and release energy that results in ionization.

Does the term "radiation" therapy refer to all treatments using ionizing radiation?

Yes. Although there are different names given to treatments, depending upon the range of wavelengths used, there are three classifications based upon the penetrating abilities of the rays.

What are the names of the three classifications of therapy treatments?

1. *Superficial therapy,* which is used for some skin lesions and is in the 85 to 140 kvp range.
2. *Intermediate therapy,* which formerly was popular in the treatment of malignancy and is usually in the 200 to 400 kvp range.
3. *Supervoltage therapy,* which is the usual form of therapy today employing voltages above 400 kvp into the mev range.

Are filters useful in attenuating the beam in therapy?

Yes. Filters are useful because they can control the resulting wavelength by eliminating the lower kvp rays. They are perhaps more important in therapy than in diagnostic radiology.

Is aluminum used as filtering material in therapy?

Yes. Aluminum is used as a filtering material but not exclusively. Because of the nature of the wavelengths and the high frequencies, it is used in combination with other metals such as tin and copper.

Is there any particular sequence of metals between target and patient?

The metal is usually placed with the tin next to the portal, then the copper, and then the aluminum next to the patient. As radiation penetrates each metal, it produces wavelength characteristic of that metal, and it is for this purpose that the aluminum is placed nearest the patient.

Is there any advantage to using a combination filter composed of these materials?

Yes. A combination filter is advantageous because of its effectiveness in filtering unwanted radiation with less reduction of output of effective radiation.

Define the term used to describe the penetration of various forms of radiation.

"Half-value layer" describes the radiation penetration. This means the amount of filtering material that is necessary to reduce the output of an x-ray beam by one half. Beams with the same half-value layer are similar in their physical and biologic effects.

What is the advantage of filtration in therapy?

As in diagnostic radiation, filtration eliminates the longer wavelengths that serve no useful purpose. Increasing the filtration increases the energy of the resulting beam. There is a point at which the output is reduced to such a low figure that treatments require too much time.

Organs and tissues of the body are classified as radiosensitive and radioresistant. Explain what this means, and give examples of each type.

Radiosensitive means susceptible to radiation, or ready responsiveness to the actions of radiation. Radioresistant means tending to resist the effects of radiation.

The following are some examples of radiosensitive areas: tumors arising from blood elements and related tissues; tumors of embryonal cell origin, normal bone marrow, and lining of the gastrointestinal tract; and tumors of the lip, skin, uterine cervix, endometrium, breast, and larynx.

Radioresistant areas include tumors of the muscles and nerves, malignant melanomas, and osteogenic sarcomas. It should be pointed out, however, that occasionally a tumor that would normally be considered radioresistant may be quite radiosensitive. It also should be emphasized that because a tumor is radiosensitive, it is not necessarily curable.

Are there statistics as to the percentage of patients treated for benign conditions?

We cannot quote any statistics, but most radiotherapists do not believe in using ionizing radiation to treat benign conditions.

Why is supervoltage radiation useful in treatment?

Supervoltage radiation causes a marked increase of radiation effect as a result of its high energy level and is more penetrating. This results in less injury to the skin and superficial tissues in relation to the amount of energy deposited in depth.

What is the difference between a linear accelerator and a cobalt therapy source?

In linear accelerators electrons are accelerated and bombard a target, which results in supervoltage x-rays, usually in the range of 2 to 6 mev. This radiation is not of a single energy but is distributed below the peak energy.

Cobalt sources employ the radioisotope cobalt 60, which decays with a five-year half-life, emitting 1.3-mev radiation. This radiation is monoenergetic and is thus compatible to the energies seen with a 2-mev linear accelerator.

What methods are used to determine measurements of the intensities of an x-ray beam at various points along its path through the body tissues?

Because of the very nature of x-rays, it is difficult to accurately determine or measure the intensity at different levels, but it has been found that by measuring the intensity in air (air dose rate) and the half-value layer (hvl) a reasonably constant measurement can be obtained.

After determining the air dose rate, we find that a reading taken at the patient's skin surface is greater than the air dose. Why is this?

Readings taken at the skin are not only measuring the air exposure but also backscatter, the secondary radiation that has been scattered back from the patient's body.

What factors determine the amount of backscatter?

Backscatter amounts are determined by the size of the treatment field, the quality of the beam of radiation, and the thickness of tissue irradiated. It should be emphasized that the relationship between backscatter and penetration is not as simple as indicated since, as the penetrating power of the primary beam increases, the secondary radiation tends to be more in the forward direction of the primary beam.

Is backscatter influenced by the source-skin distance?

No. The source-skin distance has no effect on the backscatter.

In determining depth dose, what factors should be considered?

Probably the most important factors to be considered are the amounts of radiation necessary at the predetermined depth and the methods of attaining these amounts without damaging the intervening tissues and skin. The x-ray beam does not distinguish between healthy and pathologic tissues.

What may be done to reduce the damage to the skin and healthy tissues in irradiating pathologic tissues?

The half-value layer may be increased, which will increase the percentage depth dose, or a cross-fire technique or rotational therapy may be utilized.

How is depth dose determined, since it is virtually impossible to implant instruments within the body to accurately check the intensities?

A combination of methods has been devised to check intensities, such as measuring phantoms or different depths in phantoms with known half-value layers. These phantoms usually are made of materials that absorb radiation in much the same way as living tissues. It is always known that the tissue dose rate below the surface is less than the skin dose rate because the underlying tissue is farther away from the source, and it is known that the intervening tissues will absorb some of the radiation.

In computing percentage depth dose, does the source-skin distance have any effect?

Most definitely. As the source-skin distance is increased, the percentage depth dose increases and vice versa.

Does field size affect percentage depth dose?

The percentage depth dose increases as the size of the treatment field is increased, and it decreases as the field size is reduced.

In computing dose rate to a tumor, it must be remembered that the skin dose will be greater than the tumor dose. How is this solved so that the skin will not receive an excessive dose rate?

This situation is overcome by using a greater hvl and a greater source-skin distance with a cross-fire technique. The cross-fire technique is the application of a multiportal system rather than one treatment port. Several angles around the body part to be irradiated are used. Rotational therapy is another process in which the patient is rotated in the beam so that it will strike the treatment (tumor) area from different angles.

Why must such precautions be taken if radiation is being used to treat a pathologic condition?

Such precautions must be taken because radiation effects are always destructive and deleterious both in a tumor and in its adjacent tissues. Its effects are also selective but not specifically more pronounced in malignant than in normal tissues such as skin.

Earlier it was stated that tissues were either radiosensitive or more radioresistant. Give examples of radiosensitive and radioresistant tissues.

Radiosensitive tissue would be malignant lymphoma, whereas nerve tissue is relatively radioresistant.

Is there an optimum dose rate beyond which radiation should not be given?

There is a maximum dose rate for each body area treated. Exceeding this dose rate would likely cause irreparable damage to surrounding tissues.

What amount of radiation is desired to cure a squamous cell carcinoma of the skin?

It is generally considered that the dose necessary is 6,000 r, delivered at the rate of 1,000 r per week. This will vary, depending upon the radiotherapist and the type of equipment used.

How may the amount of radiation absorbed by the body tissues be calibrated?

Readings are taken at the surface of the skin and at the exit port. The amount of radiation tallied at the exit port is subtracted from the skin dose, with the difference being the amount absorbed by the tissues.

Why is a bolus material used in 200 or 280 kvp treatments?

This is done to fill up any appreciable air space between the treatment portal and tumor, thus avoiding "hot spots" or "cold spots." The bolus acts as tissue and therefore results in a more homogeneous distribution of the radiation.

During radiotherapy, the irradiated skin becomes red. What causes this condition?

This is a reaction by the skin to radiation (erythema); it occurs occasionally and has been used as an indicator of superficial radiation response. Skin changes should be observed closely since occasionally they can become so severe they will not heal effectively.

When a large portion of the hematopoietic tissue is irradiated, how often should the white blood count be obtained during irradiation?

This should be determined by the previous count. It normally would be done once or twice weekly unless the previous count dictated otherwise, in which case it should be done more often.

How often should patients receiving radiation therapy treatments be examined by the doctor in charge for checking treatment progress?

The situation, as dictated by the nature of the treatments, reasons for treatment, and equipment used, will necessarily determine the regularity of examinations. It is important to closely observe the patients receiving radiotherapy since subtle changes may occur that would significantly alter the course of the treatment.

If an error is detected in the treatment, what should the technician do?

The technician should immediately report this error to the radiotherapist in charge. These errors should be charted in the patient's records. If time has elapsed between starting time and the time that the error is discovered, this should be reported to the therapist.

What was the first radioactive material used in treatment of carcinoma of the uterus?

Radium 226 was the first radioactive material to be used.

What is considered to be a lethal dose for humans?

This will depend on the area of the body irradiated. For total body radiation excesses of 400 r will be lethal, whereas for small areas this may cause no serious damage.

Needles used for interstitial therapy contain approximately how much radium?

The usual amount is 2 mg. radium, with the filtration of the radium capsules expressed in millimeters of platinum.

With a given machine, hvl, field size, and TSD, the dose at 8 cm. is 50 percent of the skin dose. If the skin dose is 250 r, then what is the tumor dose?

If the tumor dose is 50 percent of the skin dose, which is 250 r, then the tumor will receive 125 r.

How long does the usual therapy course take?

The entire course of therapy treatments usually requires about five weeks, although this varies with the type of lesion being treated and the form of irradiation.

What is dose fractionation?

Fractionation means dividing the dose into daily fractions. This practice is useful in protecting normal tissues from damage and also in increasing the biologic effect of the radiation in the tumor. This is the reason that most treatments take many weeks.

18 RADIOACTIVE ISOTOPES

The use of radioactive isotopes has recently reached proportions that have made it a separate specialty. Much has been learned about radiation, its properties, and methods of protection against it since Roentgen's early discoveries. Shortly after his discovery, it was noted that certain materials also act upon photographic paper, causing it to turn black or become exposed. Being aware of Roentgen's discovery and subsequent related articles, technologists believed that natural elements might also possess the ability to cause changes in certain materials. Madame Curie and her husband devoted several years to the search and were responsible for isolating radium and its many properties. The intensities by which it is measured are stated in "curies" or some fraction thereof in honor of its discoverers.

Before proceeding, perhaps it would be beneficial to review briefly the structure of matter and in this way clarify what we will be discussing in this chapter.

We have learned that all matter is made of atoms, and at one time it was believed that the atom was the smallest particle of matter. We know this is not true, and, because of Niels Bohr's work, we have learned that the atom is structured like a miniature solar system, with a nucleus and orbits around it containing electrons. The nucleus contains two kinds of particles, known as protons and neutrons. Protons have a positive charge, and neutrons carry no charge, or are neutral. The orbits, or energy levels, surrounding the nucleus contain particles known as electrons. These particles have a negative charge and revolve around the nucleus. When there are an equal number of protons and electrons in an atom, it is said to be a stable atom. If it lost one proton or electron, it would become an ion, which is unstable. Because of the laws of magnetism, the atom will remain stable unless an outside force acts upon it. The nucleus, being positively charged, exerts a certain force upon the orbits surrounding it and keeps the electrons in place. The electrons, being negative and repelling each other, will remain an equidistance apart and yet be retained in their proper shell because of the force exerted upon them by the nucleus. The neutron, although it is said to be neutral, is a complex particle consisting of a proton and an electron joined together to form a single particle.

All atoms having the same arrangement of electrons in their outer orbits will react the same chemically. The number of electrons and protons in an atom determines its atomic number. The number of protons and neutrons determines the mass number. With these facts in mind, let us proceed.

What are isotopes?

Isotopes are atoms having essentially the same number of protons and electrons but different numbers of neutrons in the nuclei. To rephrase it, an atom having the same atomic number but different mass number is an isotope.

Is it possible to separate isotopes of an element chemically and to label them?

It is normally believed that the isotopes of an element are chemically indistinguishable, but, because the atoms of different isotopes differ in mass, they react at slightly different rates.

Are radioactive isotopes found only in nature?

No. They are not found only in nature, but, in addition to the fifty different nuclides that exist in nature, there are also a great percentage that are man-made.

Are all isotopes radioactive?

No, they are not. Unstable isotopes disintegrate each second, and these disintegrations emit particles, or rays, continuously. Such an isotope is said to be radioactive. If the isotope is stable, this phenomenon does not occur and the isotope is thus not considered radioactive.

What is meant by the term "atomic disintegration"?

Atomic disintegration denotes a transformation of an individual unstable atom. This does not mean that the atom falls completely apart but that a tiny charged particle of mass, or charge, is lost from the nucleus of the atom.

In dealing with radioactive isotopes, it is desirable to know the length of time it will remain radioactive. What is this called?

This is called the half-life or the decay rate.

Define the term "half-life" or "decay rate."

Half-life refers to the amount of time necessary for a known amount of radioactive material to reduce the intensity to one half. As the process continues, the number of unstable atoms left in the isotope gradually decreases, and thus the rate at which radiation is emitted will also decrease.

Is the rate of decay the same for each radioactive isotope?

No. The rate of decay will vary for each radioactive isotope. The degree of instability will determine the rate of decay.

Since the radioactivity of a nuclide is determined by the degree of instability and in decaying it is trying to reach stability, the process appears to be a rather simple one. Is it simple?

No. It is not as simple as it appears. In decaying, the product formed may be unstable.

What is this product called?

This is called the daughter product. The daughter product in turn decays into forms that may also be unstable. This process may continue through several stages until stability is finally reached.

Is there a name for such processes?

These processes, whereby several stages are gone through to reach stability, are known as decay chain.

In the process of decaying, do radioactive isotopes emit the same form of radiation?

No. The radiation emitted by an isotope during the decay period consists of various forms of radiation. Many radioisotopes give off both particles and rays.

What types of particles or rays are emitted?

Depending upon the degree of radioactivity, a radioactive isotope will emit alpha particles and beta, gamma, and neutron radiation.

What are the differences between the types emitted?

Alpha particles are relatively slow and heavy, each carrying a double-positive electric charge. They are not very penetrating and may be stopped by a sheet of aluminum foil 0.002 inch thick.

Beta radiation is smaller and much lighter but is also classified as a particle, with each particle carrying a single, negative electric charge. The speed of these rays is much greater than that of the alpha particles and may be stopped by an inch or less of aluminum.

Gamma radiation is emitted in small units known as photons. It is most penetrating, having shorter wavelengths that are similar to x-rays. Lead is usually necessary to shield from gamma radiation.

Neutron radiation is not emitted directly by any of the common radioisotopes. It is released in large numbers in nuclear reactors. They are more penetrating than any of the other types and present a special shielding problem.

What is meant by internal conversion?

Internal conversion refers to the emission of gamma radiation. In this process the unstable nucleus transfers some of its surplus energy directly to one of the orbital electrons, expelling it from its orbit. Internal conversion and the gamma emission are two alternative ways of accomplishing the transition from a higher to a lower energy state of the same isotope.

In dealing with decay factors, what does electron capture mean?

This is the process whereby the unstable nucleus captures an orbital electron and uses it to convert a proton into a neutron. The atomic number decreases by one, but the mass number remains the same. The vacant position left in the orbit is filled by another electron from the next higher energy level.

What basic units are used to measure radioactive quantity?

The basic unit of measurement for radioactivity is the curie, which is the quantity of radioactive material reducing at the rate of 37 billion (3.7×10^{10}) disintegrations per second. Further reductions of measurements are stated as the millicurie and the microcurie.

What are the rates of disintegrations for the millicurie and the microcurie?

The millicurie's disintegration is at the rate of 37 million disintegrations per second (3.7×10^{7}), and the microcurie rate is 37,000 disintegrations per second (3.7×10^{4}). An additional unit of measurement is the millimicrocurie, which disintegrates at a rate of 3,700 disintegrations per second (3.7×10).

What is the unit of radiation dosage?

Radiation absorbed by tissues is stated in rads. The same term is used in diagnostic radiation and is defined as the absorption of 100 ergs per gram of tissue. This dose rate is dependent upon the type of radiation used, that is, alpha, gamma, or neutron.

How does the dose rate vary with types of radiation?

The roentgen and rad are, for all practical purposes, equal. The roentgen, being of the gamma ray intensity, has been given the rating of 1 rad. Alpha particles, being heavier, will create damage in tissue twenty times greater than 1 rad of x-rays. Neutrons will create damage ten times greater than x-rays. One rad of alpha rays (particles) is twenty times more destructive than x-rays; also, 1 rad of neutron rays will produce a greater tissue damage than 1 rad of x-rays. For this reason it is desirable to know the nature of the radiation when stating radiation damage.

To what does the term "specific activity" relate in dealing with radioactive nuclei?

Specific activity concerns the activity per unit mass of the source material and is expressed in curies per gram.

Define the term "rem."

Another unit of radiation dosage is rem. It is the result of the absorbed dosage in rads times the particular types of radiation—alpha, gamma, and neutron—stated as RBE. The unit of RBE dose is stated as rem.

List some of the more commonly used radioactive isotopes.

Iodine 131; gold 198; phosphorus 32; cobalt 57; radioactive vitamin B_{12}; chromium 51; and iron 59.

List briefly for what each isotope is used.

Iodine 131, probably the most widely used isotope, is used to examine the thyroid gland for disease. Gold 198 is used to control ascites or pleural effusion caused by cancer metastases in the serous surfaces of body cavities. As a diluted suspension, it is injected intravenously, and the liver collects it and then may be checked for size, shape, integrity, and position. Phosphorus 32 in solution is used for the treatment of chronic leukemia and for polycythemia vera. Cobalt 57 is used to label vitamin B_{12}, which, when given, is used as a basis for detecting pernicious anemia. Chromium 51 is used to tag red cells for diagnostic determination of red cell volume. Iron 59 is useful in the study of anemia and other disorders of red blood cells and for iron metabolism.

Since radioactive isotopes emit radiation, are rules of safe-conduct applicable as when using diagnostic x-ray and radiation therapy?

Definitely there are rules. The same precautions must be observed, and because of the half-life factor, even more rigid precautions should be followed. The AEC has established rules and regulations that must

be followed. Each isotope must be properly labeled and precautions taken to assure protection to not only the patient but also others involved or in contact with any patient having received an isotope.

Why are radioactive isotopes useful in medicine?

Isotopes sometimes offer the only alternative to surgery as a method of treatment. Because they act on tissues and because active cell growth is a characteristic of cancerous tissue, radiation in many cases may be applied to the affected area without permanently harming the surrounding healthy tissue. Unlike radiation therapy from external sources, radioactive isotopes may be taken or placed internally, and thus the radiation will be emitted from within, with the greatest intensities being at the site of the malignancies.

Are there uses other than medical for isotopes?

Isotopes are useful in a wide range of areas, and each year the list increases. They are useful in industry, agriculture, and sterilization of drugs and hospital supplies.

Are radioactive isotopes useful as therapeutic agents?

Yes. Radioactive isotopes are useful therapeutic aids, but the greater percentage of them are used as diagnostic aids. The exact percentages are vague, but it is believed that 85 percent of all isotopes currently used are used as diagnostic aids.

Why are they so useful as diagnostic aids?

Practically all organs and parts of the body may be studied by the ingestion or injection of a pharmaceutical compound composed of a radioactive atom, and the dose can be followed through the body. Certain materials will be collected by different organs, and, if a material has a known amount of radioactivity, it may then be checked with a counter at a given time interval. The normal metabolism is not disturbed by this method.

Why is radioactive cobalt useful in radiation therapy?

Radioactive cobalt is useful because it has a highly penetrating gamma radiation energy, a high output, and a reasonably long half-life. It can be readily produced in high specific activity. The target material is metallic in form and can be easily handled and encapsulated.

What are some advantages isotopes as opposed to conventional radiation equipment have for industrial applications?

Probably the most important advantage is the reduction in size of the equipment. For industrial applications the material may be enclosed in whatever is to be examined and left until the desired results are attained. To check the flow of liquids, isotopic solutions may be combined and a reading taken at a particular place and time. It may also be used to check the amount of wear to which a metal part is exposed. Foodstuff may be irradiated to prevent spoilage and for numerous other uses.

On what is the decay factor of an isotope dependent?

The direct factor determining the decay rate or half-life is the physical half-life. Physical half-life is the amount of time required for 50% of the activity or disintegrations to be lost.

Should signs be displayed in areas containing radioactive isotopes?

Yes. Signs bearing the symbol of radiation and the words "caution—radiation area" should be displayed in all areas where there is radiation of 5 to 100 mr per hour.

When an isotope is said to have a higher mev energy than another isotope, what is meant?

This refers to the isotope's having a higher half-value layer.

In dealing with isotopic solutions, what is the most practical protective method to be used?

The most practical method would be the use of lead as a protective shield.

Who exercises control over the use of radioactive isotopes?

The federal government has control over the use of radioactive isotopes and exercises it through the office of the AEC.

What is the MPD for personnel in the isotope laboratories?

The MPD, as established by the AEC, is 2.5 mr per hour. In no cases shall the dose in any thirteen-week period exceed 3 rems. No person under eighteen years of age shall be permitted to work in radiation areas.

What procedures are used to check the amount of radiation received by the workers?

There are several procedures used. Probably the best and most accurate is the wearing of film badges or ionization chambers by employees. Film badges are constructed of a small case into which a photographic film sensitive to radiation is inserted. These are checked periodically by development, and the degree of blackening on the film is read on a densitometer. The degree of blackening is a measure of the amount of radiation received by the wearer.

Ionization chambers are tubes with an electrically charged, insulated wire inside. As the wire is exposed to radioactivity, the charge is gradually depleted. These chambers may be read anytime by means of a scale on the inside of the tube and are usually worn by employees who may be exposed to a relatively high dose rate for a short period of time.

What should all measuring devices stress?

All measuring devices should stress efficiency.

Charts of the nuclides show the atomic number, atomic weight, number of neutrons in the radioactive isotope, and the number of radioactive isotopes, but they do not show one important item. What is it?

With all the information shown on a chart, it does not show if the element is natural or man-made.

REFERENCES

Radioisotopes applications, Technical bulletin RAP-1, Ottawa, Canada, 1967, Atomic Energy of Canada Ltd.

Radioisotopes handbook, Technical bulletin RP-3, Ottawa, Canada, 1961, Atomic Energy of Canada Ltd.

Radioisotopes in medicine, Chicago, June, 1966, Abbott Radio Pharmaceuticals.

Safe handling of radioactive isotopes, National Bureau of Standards Handbook No. 42, Washington, D. C., 1955.

19 EQUIPMENT MAINTENANCE

Although equipment maintenance is not directly the responsibility of the technologist, he is responsible for keeping equipment repairs to a minimum. If repairs are necessary (as they will be), the observant technologist can reduce breakdown time by having an idea as to the nature of the problem. Informing the repairman of his observations often proves invaluable and allows repairs to be made more quickly. The technologist should be cognizant of procedures to follow when differences are first noted in the performance of the equipment.

What is a penetrometer?

A penetrometer, or aluminum step wedge, is a piece of aluminum shaped like steps or a ladder. It consists of a series of aluminum bars of the same thickness and width but different length. The strips are stacked one on top of the other, with the longest being on the bottom and each succeeding step being shorter.

For what are penetrometers used?

They are useful in calibration of equipment for milliamperage and kvp. They are checked against a known density strip, and adjustments are made until the desired results are obtained.

What is a spinning top?

A spinning top, so described because it spins, is a disk of radiopaque metal about 3 inches in diameter and about $\frac{1}{8}$ inch thick. A small hole is bored in the disk near the outer edge. A center pin is inserted into the disk to allow it to spin as a top.

For what purpose is a spinning top used?

A spinning top is used to check the accuracy of timers in machines. Since machines are supplied by alternating current, the dot on the top will register any current produced as black dots. The areas exposed will correspond with the number of inpulses of exposure.

What is the purpose of a tube rating chart?

Tube rating charts supplied by the manufacturer inform the operator of the maximum permissible exposure for any combination of settings and should be rigidly followed.

When checking a timer for accuracy, what is indicated if the desired number of dots is reduced by one half?

A radiograph showing one half of the required number of dots for a given exposure is an indication that a valve tube is burned out and that the timer is now operating at half wave.

If an exposure time has been selected to show twelve dots on a test film using a spinning top and if an uneven number, either eleven or thirteen, is noted, what is likely to be the problem?

This is an indication of a faulty or inefficient timer. If too few dots are shown, it is slow; if too many are shown, it is too fast.

When exceeding tube limits established by the manufacturer, what are some of the problems likely to arise?

Probably the most serious occurrence would be pitting the target, thereby creating a gassy situation in the tube, which will impair its efficiency.

What happens when an x-ray tube is gassy?

When an x-ray tube is gassy, the milliampere meter fluctuates, usually on the high side, or the circuit breaker kicks out as soon as the exposure starts.

What are circuit breakers, and for what purpose are they used?

Circuit breakers are resistors placed into the circuit for the express purpose of disconnecting the x-ray machine from the supply source when overloading or circuit shortages occur. They may be reset and the exposure settings reduced to normal limits to allow an exposure to be made.

What is the proper method of caring for lead aprons and gloves?

When not in use, aprons should be draped over racks and gloves placed on stands provided for them. The apron racks are designed so that aprons hang properly and will not be folded or creased, causing breakage of the lead. Gloves should be placed so that they are opened to allow air to circulate inside to dry perspiration formed during use on the hands. Wearing cotton gloves and lead-lined gloves at the same time will reduce the incidence of sweating.

Should lead aprons and gloves be checked periodically for breaks?

Yes. Lead aprons and gloves should be x-rayed periodically to ascertain whether any breaks are present. If and when breaks are found, the items should be replaced.

Do cassettes require any special handling and care?

Cassettes and screens represent a considerable investment in any department and should be handled with care. The screens should be cleaned periodically, using solutions particularly made for cleaning screens. Directions for use should be followed rigidly. When commercial cleaners are not available, Ivory soap may be used. Clean sponges (2 × 2 inches and 4 × 4 inches) may be employed to apply the soap and to wipe clean, using clear water. Excessive amounts of soap and water should not be used in cleaning screens.

A film showing areas of unsharpness would likely be the result of what?

Areas of unsharpness on a film exposed in a cassette would indicate poor film-screen contact. This situation would not normally appear on cardboards or non-screen film, since the part is placed directly in contact with the film.

Does this mean that the cassette is no good and must be destroyed?

No. Usually areas of unsharpness caused by poor film-screen contact may be corrected by building up the area and inserting paper beneath the back screen to the thickness necessary to overcome the condition. This will usually require several attempts before correction is complete.

State briefly the care and maintenance of grids.

Grids, like cassettes and screens, represent a large investment, either as stationary grids or grid cassettes, and care should be taken to assure that they are not dropped or placed beneath a patient or other object that might cause them to become bent or warped. Any materials spilled on them should be cleaned away, and, when not being used, they should be placed in safe areas.

If the filament of the x-ray tube fails to light, what are the probable reasons? How could the cause be determined?

If the filament does not light, the cables can be checked at both the x-ray tube head and the transformer after turning the main switch off. This situation is usually the result of a loose wire, and, if not spotted by visual checks, a service engineer should be called.

What causes pitting of the target in the x-ray tube?

Pitting of the x-ray tube target is usually the result of overloading the focal spot by using excessive high-current valves. If the pitting is severe, the quantity of useful radiation will be diminished.

In using image intensifiers, why should caution be used in caring for the mirror?

Because of the quality of the ground optics used, it is imperative that the mirror be cleaned with materials supplied by the manufacturer or with a soft, lint-free cloth. Avoid scratches or harsh abrasives that might cause scratches.

In making an exposure it is noticed that the milliampere meter does not indicate a reading. What is likely to be the problem?

First indication would be a faulty milliampere meter if all contacts seem to be working. To check, place the open cassette on the table after darkening the room and make an exposure into the opened cassette. If the screens fluoresce, then the meter is at fault. If the screens do not fluoresce, check the cathode cable for contact.

How may you detect a broken, high-tension cable?

A broken, high-tension cable can be noticed by either visual observation and running the hand over the sheathing or by detecting the odor of burning rubber. Because of the construction of the cables, it is sometimes difficult to determine if a break does exist. Care should be taken to eliminate any sharp, sudden bends in the cables or catching them on sharp objects, which might puncture them.

A tripped circuit breaker indicates trouble where?

A tripped circuit breaker indicates trouble in the secondary or high-tension circuit.

Why are three-phase generators more efficient than full-wave generators?

The number of valve tubes is increased from four to six, and the voltage never drops to zero. Three-phase equipment utilizes more of the peak kvp and, because of this, is much more efficient.

Are short intense exposures using three-phase equipment greater or smaller than full-wave equipment regarding tube ratings?

Exposures of a short intense nature made with three-phase equipment are greater than with full-wave equipment.

Why must valve tube failure be considered when checking for a sudden density loss in radiographs?

Valve tube failure is considered because, if a valve tube is burned out, the equipment is not operating as full wave. It is now half wave, and the exposure is one half of its intensity.

How may valve tube burnout be checked?

Valve tube burnout can be checked by using a spinning top, selecting a set of exposure factors, and checking the resultant number of dots on the radiograph. Half of the required amount will indicate a burned-out valve tube.

When using a rapid film changer (Elema Schonender), should you continue with another examination without completing the run-through if the exposure is terminated prior to completion?

It is advisable to complete the entire series of film and then start a new examination by reloading the chamber. Otherwise the possibility of films jamming is increased. All new procedures should be started from the number one position.

What causes inconsistent radiographic results?

Frequently inconsistent radiographic results are caused by technical error on the part of the technician. Solutions, screens, variations in line voltage, and erratic timers are some factors affecting results, but these should be checked by the technologist.

What causes Bucky lines?

Bucky lines are the result of either the Bucky switch being out of position or the alignment of the tube and the Bucky being off. If utilizing stereo shifts, the technologist possibly can shift across the Bucky rather than with the long axis of the grid.

Why is it important in positioning the mirror of an image intensifier to place it so that light will not be reflected back into the intensifier?

Light reflected by the mirror back through the optics to the input phosphor will cause a decrease in gain over a period of time. This means that the input phosphor will not glow as brightly after exposure to refracted light.

Why is it important to clean automatic processors frequently?

Residue tends to build up on the crossover rollers during transportation of the film. This residue, if left to accumulate, will become a problem and is likely to cause jamups.

1. Secondary radiation is a product of:
   (a) overdevelopment
   (b) increase in cone size
   (c) kilovoltage
   (d) penetrameter

2. Which of the following are *not* essential to the production of radiation:
   (a) source of electrons
   (b) oscilloscope
   (c) sudden stoppage of high-speed electrons
   (d) electrons in high-speed motion

3. A moving grid is called:
   (a) Potter-Bucky diaphragm
   (b) curved grid
   (c) parallel grid
   (d) focused grid

4. Poor screen contact reduces:
   (a) density
   (b) contrast
   (c) distortion
   (d) definition

5. Exposures with an intensifying screen rather than direct exposure technique result in:
   (a) shorter exposure
   (b) longer exposure
   (c) same exposure
   (d) double exposure

6. The degree of blackening of a film by the x-ray beam is dependent upon:
   (a) speed of the film
   (b) size of the focal spot
   (c) low grid ratio
   (d) photon energy reaching the film

7. The advantage of a rotating anode tube over a stationary tube is:
   (a) larger field coverage
   (b) greater tube capacity
   (c) increase in contrast
   (d) less expensive in operating

8. A radiograph is made using an 8:1 grid. If a 16:1 grid replaces the original 8:1 grid, to maintain the same density we need to:
   (a) decrease the amount of radiation
   (b) make no change
   (c) increase the amount of radiation
   (d) use a large focal spot

9. A cone sufficient to cover a 14- × 17-inch film is used to produce a satisfactory radiograph. If a 4-inch cone is used to cone down on the gallbladder with no other factor changes, the resulting radiograph will exhibit:
   (a) mottled density
   (b) more density
   (c) less density
   (d) same density

10. When an intensifying screen continues to emit light after exposure to radiation, it is said to possess:
    (a) ionization
    (b) lag
    (c) high definition
    (d) poor contact

11. A high-ratio grid compared to a low-ratio grid will:
    (a) absorb more secondary radiation
    (b) absorb less secondary radiation
    (c) not absorb secondary radiation
    (d) absorb less primary radiation

12. Utilizing full-wave rectification, a spinning top test taken at $\frac{1}{20}$ second would indicate how many dots:
    (a) 20
    (b) 12
    (c) 4
    (d) 6

13. Which of the following is *not* one of the properties of x-rays:
    (a) travel in straight lines
    (b) cause certain substances to fluoresce
    (c) cause electrons to move at high speed
    (d) affect photographic film

14. X-rays are invisible, but their presence may be detected by:
    (a) effect on photographic film
    (b) light given off by the tube filament
    (c) movement of the kilovoltage meter
    (d) none of the above

15. The area under bombardment by electrons is known as the:
    (a) effective focal spot
    (b) actual focal spot
    (c) large focal spot
    (d) double focal spot

16. Heat units are a product of:
    (a) ma × time
    (b) kvp × ma × 2
    (c) kvp × ma × time
    (d) ma × kvp × D2

17. One of the following is true about oxygen:
    (a) has an atomic number of 1
    (b) has an atomic mass of 1
    (c) has an atomic number of 8
    (d) has an atomic number of 16
    (e) none of the above

18. The radon gas is a natural radioactive element with a half-life of about:
    (a) 4 hours
    (b) 4 days
    (c) 4 months
    (d) 4 years
    (e) 40 years

19. The white cell count is approximately:
    (a) 100 per cubic millimeter

(b) 1,000 per cubic millimeter
(c) 25,000 per cubic millimeter
(d) 5,000 per cubic millimeter
(e) 500,000 per cubic millimeter

20. One of the following is a malignant condition:
(a) arthritis
(b) tonsillitis
(c) bronchitis
(d) pernicious anemia
(e) leukemia

21. The most commonly affected valve in the adult with valvular heart disease is:
(a) tricuspid valve
(b) pulmonic valve
(c) aortic valve
(d) mitral valve
(e) ileocecal valve

22. The proton is heavier than the electron. The ratio of their masses is approximately:
(a) 2 to 1
(b) 20 to 1
(c) 200 to 1
(d) 2,000 to 1
(e) 4,000 to 1

23. In x-ray production kilovoltage and wavelength are interdependent in the following way:
(a) wavelength increases with increase of kilovoltage
(b) wavelength decreases with increase of kilovoltage
(c) wavelength is proportional to the square of the kilovoltage
(d) wavelength is proportional to the inverse square of kilovoltage
(e) wavelength is proportional to the square root of kilovoltage

24. Beta particles are also called:
(a) protons
(b) helium nucleus
(c) electrons
(d) hydrogen
(e) neutrons

25. One rad equals 100 ergs absorbed in 1 gram of:
(a) any absorber
(b) soft tissue
(c) bone
(d) water
(e) helium

26. In a therapy x-ray machine the size of field influences:
(a) output
(b) amperage
(c) backscatter
(d) kilovoltage
(e) none of the above

27. In dealing with a 250-kv x-ray therapy machine, the half-value layer is usually expressed in:
(a) millimeter of aluminum
(b) millimeter of copper
(c) millimeter of lead
(d) millimeter of gold
(e) millimeter of platinum

28. Local skin effect of radiation depends on all the following except:
(a) kilovoltage
(b) amperage
(c) half-value layer
(d) type of tumor treated
(e) filter used

29. The Pavlow position, the Twining position, and/or the "Swimmer's" view are all used to demonstrate in the lateral projection:
(a) thoracic-lumbar region
(b) lumbosacral-coccygeal region
(c) occipitocervical region
(d) cervical-lumbar region
(e) cervical-thoracic region

30. Which of the following cells is the most sensitive to radiation:
(a) epithelium
(b) mucous membrane
(c) striated muscle
(d) lymphocyte
(e) smooth muscle

31. One of the following does *not* apply to cancer:
(a) cancer is a malignant disease
(b) cancer is a benign disease
(c) cancer is often incurable
(d) cancer often produces anemia
(e) cancer is often fatal

32. Lymphosarcoma refers to:
(a) benign hyperplasia of muscle tissue
(b) malignant hyperplasia of muscle tissue
(c) benign hyperplasia of lymphoid tissue
(d) malignant hyperplasia of lymphoid tissue
(e) malignant hyperplasia of bone marrow

33. The oldest radioactive material used in intracavitary radiation therapy is:
(a) cobalt 60
(b) cesium 137
(c) radium
(d) linear accelerator
(e) iodine 131

34. Rotational x-ray therapy is not usually applied in the treatment of:
(a) carcinoma of the esophagus
(b) carcinoma of the skin
(c) carcinoma of the mediastinum
(d) carcinoma of the bladder
(e) carcinoma of the uterus

35. Which of the following radioactive materials emits only beta radiation:
    (a) cobalt 60
    (b) cesium 137
    (c) radium
    (d) phosphorus 32
    (e) iodine 131
36. Radon is a daughter product of:
    (a) radium 226
    (b) cobalt 60
    (c) phosphorus 32
    (d) iodine 131
    (e) strontium 90
37. The energy of cobalt 60 is approximately:
    (a) 0.3 mev
    (b) 0.6 mev
    (c) 0.9 mev
    (d) 1.2 mev
    (e) 1.5 mev
38. Sialography is the term applied to the injection of a radiopaque medium and the roentgenographic demonstration of which of the following:
    (a) adrenal glands
    (b) salivary glands
    (c) axillary glands
    (d) lymph glands
    (e) reproductive glands
39. Iodine 131 is usually given as:
    (a) intramuscular injection
    (b) hypodermic injection
    (c) intravenous injection
    (d) a drink, diluted in water
    (e) none of the above
40. If the intensity of radiation from an x-ray tube is 20 mr/min. at a distance of 8 feet, the intensity measured at a distance of 4 feet will be:
    (a) 5 mr/min.
    (b) 10 mr/min.
    (c) 20 mr/min.
    (d) 40 mr/min.
    (e) 80 mr/min.
41. A current of 30 milliamperes and an exposure time of 0.5 second have been used to make a given exposure. What current would be required if the exposure time were decreased to 0.05 second:
    (a) 300 milliamperes
    (b) 3000 milliamperes
    (c) 250 milliamperes
    (d) 2,500 milliamperes
    (e) 3 milliamperes
42. The correlation of knowledge by deriving certain principles is known as:
    (a) theories
    (b) scientific attitude
    (c) standardization
    (d) laws
    (e) hypothesis
43. If a force acting upon a body does not move it:
    (a) work is done
    (b) energy is expended
    (c) no work is done
    (d) energy flows from a higher level to a lower level
    (e) energy flows from a lower level to a higher level
44. The unit of work in the metric system is:
    (a) ampere
    (b) watt
    (c) ohm
    (d) joule
    (e) foot-pound
45. The smallest subdivision of a compound substance that has all the properties of the original substance is called:
    (a) photon
    (b) molecule
    (c) corpuscle
    (d) element
    (e) compound
46. The number of positive charges on the nucleus equals:
    (a) number of neutrons
    (b) atomic number
    (c) number of photons
    (d) atomic weight
    (e) number of deuterons
47. If an electron is added or removed from an atom, the atom is then called:
    (a) beta particle
    (b) little bag of marbles
    (c) deuteron
    (d) ion
    (e) proton
48. The Chasard-Lapine position best demonstrates which of the following:
    (a) ileocecal area
    (b) rectosigmoid area
    (c) diaphragmatic hernia
    (d) hepatic flexure
    (e) splenic flexure
49. In electrification by induction the kind of charge conferred on a metallic object placed in the field of a charged object is:
    (a) opposite kind
    (b) same kind
    (c) positive
    (d) negative
    (e) neutral
50. Indicate which of the following expressions does not fit with the group:
    (a) potential difference
    (b) voltage

(c) amperes
(d) emf
(e) potential drop

51. If 200 volts are applied across a resistance of 4 ohms, the current will be:
    (a) 5 milliamperes
    (b) 5 amperes
    (c) 20 amperes
    (d) 50 amperes
    (e) 512 amperes

52. To predict which way a motor armature will rotate you must use:
    (a) power rule
    (b) slide rule
    (c) right-hand rule
    (d) left-hand rule
    (e) elbow rule

53. The pair of bones that form most of the lateral wall and part of the roof of the skull are:
    (a) parietal bones
    (b) sphenoid bones
    (c) palatine bones
    (d) scapulae
    (e) occipital bones

54. The head of the pancreas lies retroperitoneally in close relationship to:
    (a) sigmoid colon
    (b) esophagus
    (c) duodenum
    (d) appendix
    (e) tonsils

55. The immovable joint that separates the frontal from the parietal bones is:
    (a) temporomandibular joint
    (b) lambdoidal suture
    (c) sagittal suture
    (d) squamoparietal suture
    (e) coronal suture

56. The mastoid process is part of the bone called:
    (a) occipital
    (b) temporal
    (c) sphenoid
    (d) zygoma
    (e) mandible

57. Insulin shock is a condition of the body when there is a need for:
    (a) insulin
    (b) saline
    (c) carbohydrate
    (d) protein

58. The process by which carbon dioxide and oxygen is exchanged in the body is known as:
    (a) apnea
    (b) anoxia

(c) Cheyne-Stokes
(d) respiration

59. If the central ray is directed perpendicular to the midline at the level of the anterior-superior iliac crest, the view taken is:
    (a) dorsal spine
    (b) AP pelvis
    (c) coned-down fifth lumbar spine
    (d) AP hip
    (e) lateral hip

60. The malleoli are used as landmarks when making a radiograph of:
    (a) AP ankle
    (b) PA knee
    (c) AP shoulder
    (d) AP elbow
    (e) AP foot

61. In radial deviation the wrist is turned:
    (a) inward
    (b) upward
    (c) downward
    (d) medially
    (e) outward

(62 through 66) Opposite each term in column A, place the number of the correct definition as listed in column B.

62. oblique
63. lateral decubitus
64. extension
65. abducted
66. dorsal

(a) rotated from true AP
(b) straightening of the part
(c) with part moved away from midline
(d) toward the back
(e) lying on the side
(f) flexion

67. All of the following statements concerning the wrist are correct except one. Select the incorrect statement.
    (a) There are eight carpal bones arranged in two rows.
    (b) The carpal bones are tightly bound together except for the navicular.
    (c) Flexion and extension can occur at the radiocarpal joint.
    (d) Flexion and extension can occur at the midcarpal joint.
    (e) The navicular acts as a connecting rod between the proximal and distal rows.

68. With a transformer whose primary has 110 turns and is connected to 110 volts, it is desired to step up the secondary voltage to 900 volts. The number of secondary turns required is:
    (a) 220
    (b) 900
    (c) 1800
    (d) does not matter

69. The use of full-wave rectification increases:
    (a) tube rating
    (b) quality of x-rays
    (c) necessary time of exposure for given milliampere and kilovoltage settings
    (d) none of the above

70. To remove an electron from the K shell of an atom, the energy of the incoming high-speed electron:
    (a) must be less than the binding energy of the K electron
    (b) must be much greater than the binding energy of the K electron
    (c) can have any value
    (d) must be at least the binding energy of the K electron

71. The wavelength of x-rays are measured in:
    (a) centimeters
    (b) millimeters
    (c) angstroms
    (d) roentgens

72. In which of the following views is an intra-oral film used:
    (a) styloid process
    (b) optic foramen
    (c) lateral nose
    (d) mandibular symphysis
    (e) pubic symphysis

73. You get the electrons to move from the cathode to the anode of an x-ray tube:
    (a) by heating the filament to higher temperatures
    (b) by having a vacuum inside the glass envelope
    (c) by putting a high voltage across the x-ray tube
    (d) by introducing a focusing cup

74. The half-value layer (hvl) is:
    (a) the thickness of material that reduces the intensity of the x-ray beam by a factor of 2
    (b) the kilovoltage used for measurement of intensity
    (c) the milliamperage that reduces the intensity by a factor of 2
    (d) the filter added on top of the x-ray tube

75. Which of the following would produce radiographs with the best detail sharpness:
    (a) detail screens
    (b) ultra-detail screens
    (c) high-speed screens
    (d) direct exposure technique

76. A film is made of the knee using a cassette and tabletop exposure. The same x-ray is made with the film in the Bucky tray; all exposure factors are the same for both exposures. The second film (Bucky) will exhibit:
    (a) more density
    (b) no change in density
    (c) greater detailed sharpness
    (d) less detailed sharpness
    (e) less density

77. Which of the following has a longer wavelength than that of x-rays:
    (a) gamma rays
    (b) all electromagnetic waves
    (c) electric waves
    (d) cosmic rays
    (e) none of these

78. Which structures are located in the left upper quadrant:
    (a) spleen, cecum, sigmoid, fundus
    (b) spleen, left adrenal, fundus, splenic flexure
    (c) duodenal bulb, splenic flexure, left kidney
    (d) hepatic flexure, left adrenal, liver, gallbladder

79. The zygomatic arch includes part, or all, of the:
    (a) temporal bone
    (b) maxilla
    (c) frontal bone
    (d) sphenoid bone

80. A type of radiation called secondary (scattered) would be that which:
    (a) emerges from the tube and reaches the patient
    (b) emerges from the patient and reaches the film
    (c) scatters on contact with the patient
    (d) controls image distortion

81. Short-scale contrast is defined by:
    (a) more contrast
    (b) less contrast
    (c) product of high kilovoltage
    (d) product of secondary radiation

82. Iodine is a:
    (a) metal
    (b) sugar
    (c) halogen
    (d) starch
    (e) amino acid

83. A polyp of the colon is a form of:
    (a) tumor
    (b) infection
    (c) cancer
    (d) fungus
    (e) ulceration

84. An angiogram shows the:
    (a) jejunum
    (b) ureters
    (c) bile ducts

(d) lymph nodes
(e) blood vessels

85. A sialogram is an examination of the:
    (a) ear
    (b) eye
    (c) mouth
    (d) salivary gland
    (e) T tube

Note: Please read carefully.

A radiograph has been taken of a lateral skull. The film is entirely satisfactory. Having been properly processed, it is placed on a view box to be used as a standard for comparison with a series of films to be taken of the same skull. In each of the ensuing exposures only one factor or condition is changed from the original.

Each of the resulting radiographs is to be compared with the original in some respects. You are to determine from your own knowledge in what regard or regards each of the experimental films will differ. A 1.0-mm. focal spot. Intensifying screens. Develop five minutes at 68° F. Bucky diaphragm 8 to 1. Cone cover 10- × 12-inch film. Forty-inch anode film distance, 100 ma., 0.5 second, 65 kvp.

The above information is to be used in answering questions 86 through 89 only.

86. Twenty-four-hour development would increase:
    (a) detail
    (b) density
    (c) contrast
    (d) magnification and/or distortion
87. Increased object-film distance would primarily decrease:
    (a) detail
    (b) density
    (c) contrast
    (d) magnification
88. Three-inch mastoid cone would increase:
    (a) density
    (b) contrast
    (c) detail visability
    (d) magnification and/or distortion
89. Added filtration of 3 mm. Al would increase:
    (a) detail
    (b) density
    (c) magnification and/or distortion
    (d) contrast
90. Tissue opacity must be considered because:
    (a) the more dense the tissue, the greater the absorption of radiation
    (b) the more dense the tissue, the less absorption and the greater the amount of remnant radiation reaching the film

(c) the more dense the tissue, the greater the absorption, the less remnant radiation reaching the film
(d) tissue opacity is the physician's area of consideration; your only interest or responsibility is to measure the part and select factors based only on centimeter measurement
(e) there are variations in temperatures of developing solutions

91. An x-ray tube has a heat storage capacity of 155,000 ahu. How many films in rapid succession can you make before exceeding the capacity of the tube when using the following exposure factors: 300 ma, 35 kvp, four seconds, 30-inch distance:
    (a) two
    (b) three
    (c) four
    (d) five
92. A criteria for attaining satisfactory radiographic quality would be:
    (a) contrast should be such that differentiation between densities or details can be readily made
    (b) always use short-scale contrast
    (c) always use long-scale contrast
    (d) contrast choice is unimportant in radiographic quality
93. Which view best shows the condition of the ankle mortice:
    (a) anteroposterior and lateral ankle
    (b) anteroposterior ankle with central ray directed to the ankle mortise at angles of 10, 20, 30, and 40 degrees
    (c) anteroposterior ankle with foot in inversion
    (d) true lateral of ankle joint
94. To show the neck of the femur in a true anatomic position:
    (a) feet are in internal rotation
    (b) feet are in external rotation
    (c) feet are in neutral position
    (d) knees are flexed
95. Spondylolisthesis is a condition arising from a forward displacement of one vertebra upon another. What views are indicated:
    (a) oblique views of lumbar spine
    (b) a satisfactory lateral view
    (c) scoliosis series
    (d) spot film of D-12
96. When doing oblique views of the cervical spine in the anterior oblique position:
    (a) the foramina disclosed are on the side nearest the film
    (b) no foramina are disclosed
    (c) you must use a 36-inch focal-film distance

(d) the foramina disclosed are on the side nearest the tube

97. What view will show a fracture of noncalcified costal cartilage to the best advantage:
 (a) LAO
 (b) LPO
 (c) PA chest
 (d) none of the above

98. With the patient in the supine position, the radiographic baseline is placed parallel to the film. This is called:
 (a) posteroanterior position
 (b) Towne position
 (c) verticosubmental position
 (d) reverse Towne position
 (e) submentovertical position

99. The sella turcica may best be localized for spot films:
 (a) 1 inch above and 2 inches posterior to auditory meatus
 (b) 1 inch above and 1 inch anterior to auditory meatus
 (c) 2 inches above and 2 inches posterior to auditory meatus
 (d) 2 inches above and 2 inches anterior to auditory meatus
 (e) 1 inch superior and 1 inch inferior to auditory meatus

100. The constant relation between intensity of radiation and time of exposure in producing a given degree of blackening is:
 (a) sensitivity
 (b) film speed
 (c) inverse logarithm of the hydrogen ion concentration
 (d) reciprocity
 (e) inverse logarithm of the ratio of transmitted to incident light on the film

101. If the medial plane, radiographic base line, and central x-ray beam are all perpendicular to the x-ray table, and the interorbital line and coronal plane are parallel to the table, the skull is positioned in a true (choose one of the following):
 (a) posteroanterior view
 (b) lateral view
 (c) reverse Towne view
 (d) Mayer view
 (e) base view

102. Which of the following positions for the pars petrosa requires the skull rotated 45 degrees toward the film and the tube angled 45 degrees toward the feet:
 (a) Stenver position
 (b) Schuller position
 (c) Mayer position
 (d) Hickey position
 (e) Granger position

103. To obtain an unobstructed view of the petrous apex, semicircular canals, vestibule, and cochlea, together with the internal auditory meatus and canals, which of the following views must be used:
 (a) Hickey view
 (b) Law view
 (c) Mayer view
 (d) attic view
 (e) Stenver view

104. The size and shape of the spleen, liver, and kidneys are best visualized in which of the following views of the abdomen:
 (a) right anterior oblique
 (b) anterior and posterior supine view
 (c) lateral view
 (d) anteroposterior view with x-ray beam horizontal
 (e) Waters view

105. Sialography is the term applied to the roentgenographic demonstration with the injection of a radiopaque medium of the:
 (a) salivary glands
 (b) adrenal glands
 (c) axillary glands
 (d) lymph glands
 (e) reproductive glands

106. The superior vena cava transmits blood:
 (a) from the lungs to the heart
 (b) from the heart to the lungs
 (c) from the head and arms to the heart
 (d) from the bowel to the liver
 (e) from the fetus to the placenta

107. Which of the following studies are performed by an intravenous injection of contrast material:
 (a) nephrotomography
 (b) retrograde pyelography
 (c) cystourethrography
 (d) retroperitoneal air insufflation
 (e) renal arteriography

108. When critiquing a radiograph for its medical legal application, we look for:
 (a) correct choice of radiographic technique
 (b) proper and adequate illumination
 (c) proper identification and radiation protection
 (d) retroperitoneal air insufflation
 (e) renal arteriography

109. The criterion for attaining satisfactory radiographic quality is:
 (a) all portions of the image should have silver deposits
 (b) short scale of contrast should be used
 (c) collimator should be opened to its fullest extent
 (d) detail should not be obscured by fog

110. What is the purpose of celiac angiography:

(a) It is usually performed to demonstrate circulation to the colon.

(b) It is performed only with the use of a single straight catheter.

(c) It never results in demonstration of the portal vein.

(d) It is never performed using a pressure injector.

(e) It is to demonstrate the vessels of the liver, spleen, pancreas, and stomach.

111. Compton absorption process is important in absorption of x-rays of:
(a) low energy
(b) high energy
(c) conventional x-ray therapy energy
(d) not important at all

112. An x-ray therapy department may possess all the following equipment except:
(a) 250-kv x-ray machine
(b) 400-kv x-ray machine
(c) cobalt 60 unit
(d) cesium 137 machine
(e) phosphorus 32 machine

113. The film emulsion is composed of:
(a) potassium bromide
(b) silver plus gelatin
(c) silver halide plus gelatin
(d) Mylar
(e) potassium hydroxide

114. For maximum speed and contrast, films in 68° developer should be developed about:
(a) three minutes
(b) five minutes
(c) four minutes
(d) four and one half minutes

115. A foreign particle disease of the lung, pneumoconiosis, is:
(a) pneumococcus
(b) streptococcus
(c) filariasis
(d) lung flukes
(e) silicosis

116. Prognosis is defined as:
(a) the science of pathology
(b) forecast of the probable result of disease
(c) lowered pragmatism
(d) method of examination
(e) detailed program of treatment

117. The radiographic tube used for pediatric radiography should have a high output with short exposures because:
(a) short exposures of $\frac{1}{30}$ to $\frac{1}{60}$ second are necessary to eliminate motion caused by respiration
(b) poor contrast will otherwise result
(c) radiation dose will be higher for long than for short exposures

118. Three projections are taken when there is a question of acute abdominal pain. They are recumbent anteroposterior, lateral, and:
(a) anteroposterior inverted view
(b) lateral inverted view
(c) lateral erect view
(d) anteroposterior erect view
(e) right lateral decubitus

119. Light reflected from the mirror of the image intensifier, back through the optics to the input phosphor:
(a) has no effect
(b) produces a bright spot
(c) causes a decrease in gain over a period of time
(d) causes an increase in gain over a period of time

120. Three-phase generators are more efficient than are full-wave because:
(a) voltage never drops to zero
(b) cables are larger
(c) there is higher milliamperage at longer exposures
(d) they are more expensive to purchase

121. A half-wave generator at $\frac{1}{20}$ second will produce how many "dots" on a film using a spinning top:
(a) 6
(b) 3
(c) 12
(d) 11

122. The hyoid bone is attached to the mandible by one of the following muscles:
(a) digastric muscle
(b) omohyoid muscle
(c) stylohyoid muscle
(d) hyoglossus muscle

123. The chain of command in the x-ray department is as follows:
(a) radiologist-resident radiologist-staff technician-chief technician-student
(b) radiologist-chief technician-resident-staff technician-student
(c) radiologist-resident-chief technician-student-staff technician
(d) radiologist-resident-chief technician-staff technician-student
(e) radiologist-student-resident-chief technician-staff technician

124. Naturally radioactive elements are:
(a) high atomic number elements
(b) those liberating only gamma radiation
(c) low atomic number elements
(d) those liberating only beta radiation
(e) elements in a gaseous state only

125. To determine the area of coverage afforded

by a particular cone, the following formula is used:

$$\frac{\text{FFD} \times \text{diameter of lower edge of cone}}{\text{distance from FS to lower edge of cone}}$$

If the diameter of the lower edge of the cone is 3 inches, the distance from the focal spot to the lower edge of the cone is 15 inches, and the FFD is 30 inches, the area covered by the cone will be:
(a) 10 inches
(b) 6 inches
(c) 18 inches
(d) 4 inches

126. The ma required for a given radiographic density is:
(a) directly proportional to the time
(b) directly proportional to the time squared
(c) inversely proportional to the time
(d) inversely proportional to the time squared

127. Two isotopes of the same element have:
(a) different numbers of protons
(b) same mass number
(c) different atomic weights
(d) same proportion of neutrons and protons
(e) same total number of neutrons and protons

128. The atomic weight of an atom is the:
(a) number of protons in the nucleus
(b) number of electrons
(c) number of neutrons
(d) number of protons and neutrons in the nucleus
(e) number of protons and electrons

129. A radiation intensity of 36r is recorded at a FFD of 36 inches. We wish to reduce the intensity to 9r. What new distance will be required:
(a) 72 inches
(b) 18 inches
(c) 46 inches
(d) 9 inches

130. Alpha particles are:
(a) nucleus of a helium atom
(b) helium atom minus the electrons and neutrons
(c) smaller than beta particles
(d) lighter than beta particles
(e) more penetrating than beta particles

131. An exposure time of one second had been employed at an FFD of 40 inches. It is desired to reduce the time to 0.5 second. What new distance is required to maintain the same quality radiograph:
(a) 56 inches

(b) 28 inches
(c) 44 inches
(d) 38 inches

132. Gamma rays are:
(a) high-speed electrons emitted by radioactive nuclei
(b) electromagnetic radiations coming from atomic nuclei
(c) produced when electrons jump between electron orbits in atoms
(d) emitted by all radioisotopes

133. A routine chest film is taken using a 72-inch FFD, 10 mas at 70 kvp. If the distance is reduced to 56-inch FFD, what mas should be used to obtain the same quality results:
(a) 16 mas
(b) 12 mas
(c) 9 mas
(d) 6 mas

134. A microcurie is:
(a) 1,000 curies
(b) 1,000 millicuries
(c) 1/100 millicurie
(d) 1/1,000 millicurie
(e) 1/1,000 curie

135. Changing from a 1-mm. focal spot to 0.05-mm. focal spot would increase:
(a) density
(b) detail
(c) contrast
(d) magnification/distortion

136. The correct formula for computing anode heat units is:
(a) kvp × mas × fs = ahu
(b) tfd × ma × time = ahu
(c) 60 cycles × kvp × time = ahu
(d) kvp × ma × time = ahu

137. In radiologic technology a film critique may be considered as:
(a) an overexposed film
(b) excellent contrast and density
(c) technical evaluation of a radiograph
(d) proper and adequate radiographic technique

138. Radioactive cobalt is useful in medical therapy because:
(a) it has a short half-life
(b) it emits energetic beta rays
(c) it is a long-lived gamma ray emitter
(d) it is concentrated in brain tumors
(e) it is easy to shield against its radiations

139. One of the following methods is *never* used to remove radioactive contamination:
(a) washing with a detergent
(b) soaking in a nonradioactive solution of the contaminant
(c) treatment with dilute acids

(d) storing for several half-lives

(e) boiling in water

140. It is necessary to wear rubber gloves when:
    (a) handling a bottle of urine from a patient who has received isotope treatment for thyroid cancer
    (b) transferring radioactive samples to a counter
    (c) measuring the thyroid uptake of a patient
    (d) pouring a radioactive drink of 5 microcuries for thyroid uptake
    (e) handling a sealed beta applicator for treatment of skin cancer

141. All artifacts fall into which category:
    (a) poor radiograph density
    (b) areas of increased or decreased density
    (c) long scale of radiographic contrast
    (d) radiation, white, or safelight fog

142. Bones have definite structure directly relating to specific functions. Check the following function that is incorrect:
    (a) protection
    (b) supply lymph fluid
    (c) support and framework
    (d) levers

143. Which of the following is electromagnetic radiation:
    (a) beta rays
    (b) gamma rays
    (c) alpha rays
    (d) neutron beam
    (e) proton beam

144. Which of the following has the smallest size:
    (a) electron
    (b) neutron
    (c) gamma ray
    (d) alpha particle
    (e) beta particles

145. Which of the following types of electromagnetic radiation has the shortest wavelength:
    (a) radio waves
    (b) infrared waves
    (c) x-rays
    (d) visible light
    (e) ultraviolet waves

146. Only relatively heavy nuclides (high Z) decay with the emission of:
    (a) neutrons
    (b) positrons
    (c) electrons
    (d) alpha particles
    (e) gamma rays

147. The measure of radiation intensity in air is the:
    (a) rad
    (b) RBE

(c) Rutherford

(d) rem

(e) roentgen

148. Ionization chambers depend upon the ———— to enable them to measure radiation intensity.
    (a) ionization effect
    (b) current
    (c) voltage
    (d) power
    (e) electronic components

149. The decay factor for any isotope depends directly on the:
    (a) half-value layer
    (b) type of radiation emitted
    (c) biologic half-life
    (d) physical half-life
    (e) intensity

150. The radiation symbol with the words "Caution: Radiation Area" should be displayed where:
    (a) there is radiation of 100 mr./hr. or above
    (b) there is radiation of 5 mr/hr. to 100 mr/hr.
    (c) there is radiation of 0.3 mr/hr.
    (d) there is radiation of 0.2 mr/hr.
    (e) there is radiation of 0.1 mr/hr.

151. Of the following protective methods, which is usually the most practical for isotopic solutions used in medical laboratories:
    (a) distance
    (b) lead
    (c) glass
    (d) metal
    (e) concrete

152. A roentgen is a:
    (a) biologic term
    (b) physical term
    (c) measure of radiation intensity
    (d) measure of radiation quality
    (e) measure of ionization

153. A film badge depends on the ———— principle for detecting radiation intensity.
    (a) electronic
    (b) photographic
    (c) filtration
    (d) equilibrium
    (e) quantity

154. Dose meters differ from dose rate meters by:
    (a) energy
    (b) intensity
    (c) time
    (d) quality
    (e) quantity

155. The federal government control over the use of isotopes is exercised by the:

(a) FCC
(b) CAB
(c) ICC
(d) AEC
(e) ABC

156. An electroscope is a device to:
(a) indicate the presence of radiation
(b) charge material by induction
(c) charge objects by contact
(d) store electric charge
(e) dissipate charge

157. The largest use of medical isotopes is for:
(a) treatment
(b) diagnosis
(c) prognosis
(d) prophylaxis
(e) research

158. The chart of the nuclides does not show one of the following:
(a) atomic number
(b) atomic weight
(c) number of radioactive isotopes
(d) whether an element is natural or man-made
(e) number of neutrons in radioactive isotopes

159. The thoracic duct conveys:
(a) blood to the thoracic wall
(b) air from the larynx to the lungs
(c) blood from the right ventricle to the lungs
(d) lymph from the bowel to the liver
(e) lymph from lymph nodes to the subclavian vein

160. The principle used in the moving coil galvanometer is the:
(a) principle of mutual induction
(b) principle of self-induction with low r in parallel measures current
(c) principle of electrostatic induction
(d) motor principle
(e) generator principle

161. In radiographic quality, contrast is directly controlled by:
(a) ma
(b) time
(c) tfd
(d) kvp

162. In radiographic quality densities are directly controlled by:
(a) ofd
(b) mas and tfd
(c) screen contact
(d) age of patient

163. The type of radiation called primary is:
(a) that which emerges from the tube and reaches the patient

(b) that which emerges from the patient and reaches the film
(c) that which is controlled by mas
(d) that which is controlled and cut off by cones

164. A definition of radiographic contrast would be the:
(a) degree of blackening
(b) relationship between one density and another
(c) amount of visible detail
(d) amount of geometric detail

165. High-ratio grids serve what function in the control of radiographic quality:
(a) prevent distortion
(b) filter out 100 percent of the remnant radiation
(c) move back and forth under the x-ray table
(d) filter out a high degree of scattered radiation
(e) expense or cost

166. Extreme overheating of an x-ray tube will result in:
(a) heavy, dense films
(b) light, gray films
(c) shortened x-ray tube life
(d) rapid film processing because you have overexposed and underdeveloped
(e) skin burns

167. Visual detail may be partially obliterated by:
(a) poor screen-film contact
(b) too great a tube-to-film distance causing magnification
(c) too great a distance between the cathode and the anode of the x-ray tube
(d) decreasing kvp and increasing mas in proper ratio
(e) industrial film

168. In the examination of the petrous apices, which of the following is not used:
(a) lordotic view
(b) Towne view
(c) Stenvers view
(d) Law projection
(e) all of the above

169. The foramen magnum can best be seen in the:
(a) posteroanterior view of skull
(b) anteroposterior view of skull
(c) Towne view of skull
(d) Waters view of skull
(e) Caldwell view of skull

170. In the Waters position for the maxillary sinuses, the radiographic base line forms what angle with the plane of the film:
(a) 25 degrees

(b) 27 degrees
(c) 30 degrees
(d) 35 degrees
(e) 37 degrees

171. The Law position is used for an examination of the:
    (a) foramen ovale
    (b) foramen magnum
    (c) petrous tips
    (d) mastoid air cells
    (e) foramen spinosum

172. In the true Law position the central ray is directed:
    (a) 15 degrees toward the feet, 15 degrees superiorly
    (b) 15 degrees toward the feet, 15 degrees toward the face
    (c) 15 degrees toward the head, 15 degrees toward the face
    (d) 15 degrees toward the head, 15 degrees toward the base of skull
    (e) 15 degrees toward the feet, 15 degrees posteriorly

173. With the patient lying so that the median plane is parallel with the tabletop and the interpupillary line is perpendicular to the film, the view to be taken is:
    (a) posteroanterior of skull
    (b) basal of skull
    (c) occipital of skull
    (d) lateral of skull
    (e) anteroposterior of skull

174. Which of the following is radiographed in the upright position to demonstrate fluid levels:
    (a) carotid artery
    (b) spinosum ovale
    (c) mandibular menti
    (d) parotid duct
    (e) sinuses

175. The amount of tube shift required in making stereoscopic radiographs is determined by:
    (a) object-film distance
    (b) milliampere-seconds used
    (c) kilovoltage used
    (d) target-film distance
    (e) type of x-ray tube used

176. A line drawn between the pupils of the eye is called:
    (a) Reid's base line
    (b) interpupillary line
    (c) canthomeatal line
    (d) orbitomeatal line
    (e) glabellomeatal line

177. The Caldwell position has the central ray angled:
    (a) 23 degrees to feet

(b) 20 degrees to face
(c) 15 degrees to face
(d) 15 degrees to feet
(e) 10 degrees to feet

178. In the examination of the gallbladder, a lateral decubitus view is usually taken to show:
    (a) mobility of gallbladder
    (b) layering of gallstones
    (c) dye content of stone
    (d) increased density of gallbladder
    (e) decreased density of gallbladder

179. A danger sign in iodine reaction is:
    (a) sneezing
    (b) flushing
    (c) itching of the throat
    (d) cough
    (e) anxiety

180. The drug for intravenous cholangiograms is:
    (a) Lipiodal
    (b) barium
    (c) Gastrografin
    (d) Cholografin
    (e) Pantopaque

181. The drug for myelogram is:
    (a) Pantopaque
    (b) Gastrografin
    (c) Cholografin
    (d) barium
    (e) Hypaque

182. A barium enema should not be performed in cases of:
    (a) bleeding
    (b) acute appendicitis
    (c) tuberculosis
    (d) pyelotis
    (e) asthma

183. Duodenal ulcers are a form of:
    (a) cancer
    (b) infection
    (c) mucosal erosion
    (d) polyp
    (e) tuberculosis

184. Intravenous gallbladder dye must be given:
    (a) rapidly
    (b) in divided doses
    (c) slowly
    (d) under pressure

185. An air encephalogram has the needle inserted through the:
    (a) skull
    (b) neck
    (c) eye
    (d) lumbar spine
    (e) sacrum

186. Check below the word that does *not* apply to the construction of a grid:

(a) grid ratio
(b) radius
(c) linear
(d) amplitude

187. A *decrease* in grid ratio would result in:
(a) no change in exposure
(b) increase in exposure
(c) decrease in exposure
(d) out of focus exposure

188. A Potter-Bucky diaphragm in known as a:
(a) high-ratio grid
(b) grid without a ratio or radius
(c) grid in motion during exposure
(d) special type of a cone

189. To show subluxation of the acromioclavicular joints, which of the following views should be used:
(a) anteroposterior of both shoulders
(b) axial of both shoulders
(c) anteroposterior of both shoulders with weight bearing
(d) open- and closed-mouth views
(e) transperineal views

190. To x-ray the longitudinal arches for "flat feet," in which of the following positions must the patient be placed:
(a) sitting
(b) standing
(c) prone
(d) supine
(e) "frog" position

191. Which of the following parts would you x-ray if a patient came to your department with a requisition questioning a trimalleolar fracture:
(a) facial bones
(b) acoustic meatus
(c) knee
(d) ankle
(e) upper and lower teeth

192. What view best demonstrates the intercondyloid notch or space:
(a) anteroposterior view of mandible
(b) "tunnel" view of knee
(c) transthoracic view
(d) oblique views of patella
(e) lateral obliques of jaw

193. The anteroposterior projection of the cervical spine through the open mouth will demonstrate which of the following:
(a) C-7
(b) upper and lower molars
(c) atlas, axis, and odontoid process
(d) foramen magnum
(e) both tonsils

194. Why is it sometimes necessary to have the patient "breathe" during the exposure for a lateral thoracic spine:
(a) to blur out the vertebra
(b) to demonstrate the movement of the diaphragm
(c) to blur out the superimposed ribs
(d) to shorten the exposure
(e) to make the patient comfortable

195. To determine motion in the area of a spinal fusion of the lumbar sacral spine, which of the following views is indicated:
(a) lateral recumbent
(b) lateral upright
(c) lateral horizontal
(d) lateral in flexion and extension
(e) anteroposterior with legs flexed and extended

196. In the anteroposterior oblique views of the sacroiliac joints, the affected side must be:
(a) away from the film
(b) toward the film
(c) parallel to the film
(d) 60 degrees toward the film

197. The shallow breathing technique is used on which of the following examinations:
(a) lateral view of neck
(b) lateral view of sternum
(c) lateral chest
(d) oblique view of sternum
(e) none of the above

198. To demonstrate a fracture in the axillary portion of the ribs, which of the following positions are best:
(a) oblique
(b) posteroanterior
(c) lateral
(d) anteroposterior
(e) superoinferior

199. To visualize the ribs below the diaphragm to best advantage, the patient must be instructed to:
(a) take in a deep breath and hold it
(b) exhale fully and hold it
(c) say "E"
(d) breathe normally
(e) hold his breath for 10 seconds

200. To demonstrate an unobstructed view of the apices and also interlobar effusions, which of the following views would you take:
(a) posteroanterior of chest
(b) right anterior oblique of chest
(c) anteroposterior lordotic of chest
(d) lateral decubitus of chest
(e) dorsal decubitus of chest

SIMULATED REGISTRY EXAMINATION I ANSWER SHEET

1.	c	26.	c	51.	d	76.	e	101.	a	126.	c	151.	b	176.	b
2.	b	27.	b	52.	c	77.	c	102.	c	127.	c	152.	c	177.	a
3.	a	28.	d	53.	a	78.	b	103.	e	128.	d	153.	b	178.	b
4.	d	29.	e	54.	c	79.	a	104.	b	129.	a	154.	c	179.	c
5.	a	30.	d	55.	e	80.	c	105.	a	130.	a	155.	d	180.	d
6.	d	31.	b	56.	b	81.	a	106.	c	131.	b	156.	a	181.	a
7.	b	32.	d	57.	c	82.	c	107.	a	132.	b	157.	e	182.	b
8.	c	33.	c	58.	d	83.	a	108.	c	133.	d	158.	d	183.	c
9.	c	34.	b	59.	c	84.	e	109.	a	134.	d	159.	e	184.	c
10.	b	35.	d	60.	a	85.	d	110.	e	135.	b	160.	d	185.	d
11.	a	36.	a	61.	e	86.	b	111.	c	136.	b	161.	d	186.	d
12.	d	37.	d	62.	a	87.	a	112.	e	137.	b	162.	b	187.	c
13.	c	38.	b	63.	e	88.	c	113.	c	138.	c	163.	a	188.	c
14.	a	39.	d	64.	b	89.	d	114.	b	139.	e	164.	b	189.	c
15.	b	40.	e	65.	c	90.	c	115.	e	140.	a	165.	d	190.	b
16.	c	41.	a	66.	d	91.	b	116.	b	141.	c	166.	c	191.	d
17.	c	42.	d	67.	b	92.	a	117.	a	142.	b	167.	a	192.	b
18.	b	43.	c	68.	b	93.	c	118.	d	143.	b	168.	a	193.	c
19.	d	44.	d	69.	a	94.	a	119.	c	144.	a	169.	c	194.	c
20.	e	45.	b	70.	d	95.	b	120.	a	145.	c	170.	e	195.	d
21.	d	46.	b	71.	c	96.	d	121.	b	146.	d	171.	d	196.	b
22.	d	47.	d	72.	d	97.	d	122.	a	147.	e	172.	b	197.	d
23.	b	48.	b	73.	c	98.	e	123.	d	148.	a	173.	d	198.	a
24.	c	49.	a	74.	a	99.	b	124.	a	149.	d	174.	e	199.	b
25.	a	50.	c	75.	d	100.	d	125.	b	150.	b	175.	d	200.	c

SIMULATED REGISTRY EXAMINATION II

1. A line between the external auditory meatus and the outer canthus of the eye is called the:
   (a) acanthomeatal line
   (b) radiographic base line
   (c) infraorbitomeatal line
   (d) supraorbitomeatal line

2. The most satisfactory oblique projection of the lumbar vertebrae may be accomplished by rotating the body from the true lateral so that the coronal plane forms an angle with the table top at:
   (a) 35 degrees
   (b) 45 degrees
   (c) 15 degrees
   (d) 25 degrees

3. Which of the following projections would *best* demonstrate the zygomatic arches:
   (a) posteroanterior
   (b) anteroposterior
   (c) lateral
   (d) submentovertical

4. Minor degrees of overloading of the tube will result in:
   (a) defective ohmmeter
   (b) pitting of target
   (c) buildup of filtration on tube window
   (d) filament burnout

5. A timer measuring impulses of alternating current starting at zero and terminating at zero is a:
   (a) mechanical timer
   (b) synchronous timer
   (c) Gieger counter
   (d) impulse timer

6. In radiography of the sacrum in the antero-posterior position, the central ray is directed:
   (a) perpendicular to the film
   (b) cephalad
   (c) caudad
   (d) to a point 2 inches above the superior iliac spine

7. Three-phase equipment utilizes more of the peak kvp than does conventional full-wave (four-valve tube) equipment. The percentage of efficiency of three-phase equipment is:
   (a) 95
   (b) 70
   (c) 80
   (d) 100

8. What type of generator makes more effective use of the current:
   (a) self-rectified
   (b) full-wave four-valve
   (c) half-wave
   (d) six-valve

9. Three-phase generators are more efficient than full-wave because:
   (a) the voltage never drops to zero
   (b) the cables are larger
   (c) there is higher ma at larger exposures
   (d) they are more expensive to purchase

10. The secondary coil of a transformer will produce:
    (a) alternating current always
    (b) direct current always
    (c) alternating current part of the time and direct current part of the time
    (d) always a higher voltage than the primary coil
    (e) more power than is put into the primary

11. The unit of electric power is the watt. Which of the following is correct:
    (a) watts = amperes × ohms
    (b) watts = volts/amperes
    (c) watts = amperes/volts
    (d) watts = volts × amperes
    (e) watts = ohms/volts

12. In the dorsoplantar projection of the foot, the thickness of the part is measured at the:
    (a) proximal end of the third metatarsal
    (b) talonavicular joint
    (c) distal end of the metatarsals
    (d) base of the distal phalanges

13. In positioning for a true lateral of the skull, with the central ray perpendicular to the film, the median plane should be:
    (a) at an angle of 15 degrees with the film
    (b) at an angle of 15 degrees with the central ray
    (c) perpendicular to the film
    (d) parallel with the film

14. X-rays result from the bombardment of a suitable target by high-speed:
    (a) atoms
    (b) electrons
    (c) neutrons
    (d) ions
    (e) protons

15. The characteristic radiation from an x-ray tube target is produced by electrons in the target atoms that:
    (a) move from the K shell to one of the outer electron shells
    (b) move from the L shell to one of the outer shells
    (c) move from the K shell to the nucleus
    (d) move from an outer electron shell to the L shell
    (e) move from outer electron shell to the K shell

16. Sweet's localizer is likely to be used in an examination of the:

(a) sinuses
(b) eye
(c) gastrointestinal tract
(d) bladder

17. If an x-ray tube is used with a smaller focal spot, the penumbra will be:
(a) decreased
(b) increased
(c) the same
(d) darker

18. The efficiency of a grid is strongly related to the:
(a) grid ratio
(b) grid radius
(c) interspacing material
(d) lines per inch

19. The most dorsally situated portion of a typical vertebra is called the:
(a) body
(b) odontoid
(c) pedicle
(d) spinous process
(e) facet

20. The three main components of the sternum are the body, xiphoid, and:
(a) acromion
(b) glenoid
(c) manubrium
(d) pedicle
(e) talus

21. A curve representing the relation between the energy absorbed by a film during exposure and the resultant density is the:
(a) sine wave
(b) characteristive curve
(c) photographic effect
(d) attenuation curve

22. Radiographic contrast is *directly* influenced by the:
(a) milliamperage
(b) milliampere-seconds
(c) kilovoltage
(d) time

23. A radiograph is made at 85 kvp and 25 mas without a grid. If an 8:1 ratio grid is added, the mas required would then be:
(a) 25
(b) 100
(c) 150
(d) 300

24. An exposure is made at 40 inches focal-film distance using 100 mas. At 60 inches the exposure required would be:
(a) 50 mas
(b) 150 mas
(c) 225 mas
(d) 300 mas

25. The sharpness of detail in a radiograph is decreased by use of:
(a) large focal spot
(b) a grid
(c) a decrease of 10 kvp
(d) increased filtration

26. The function of contrast in a radiographic film is to:
(a) decrease latitude
(b) increase the average density
(c) provide background density
(d) make detail visible

27. The sharpness of detail is primarily dependent on a screen's:
(a) intensification factor
(b) resolving power
(c) static resistance
(d) spectral emission

28. In body section radiography a thin section of the body may be obtained by:
(a) a short amplitude and a long target-film distance
(b) a long amplitude and a short target-film distance
(c) a short amplitude and a short target-film distance
(d) a long amplitude and a long target-film distance

29. The chief advantage of employing high kvp technique (over 100 kvp) in radiography is to:
(a) preserve tube life
(b) increase latitude
(c) increase contrast
(d) decrease ma

30. The innominate bone is comprised of the pubis, ilium, and:
(a) ileum
(b) glenoid
(c) ischium
(d) femur
(e) sacrum

31. The odontoid process will be visualized in the:
(a) lateral view of the tarsus
(b) oblique view of the mandible
(c) open-mouth view of the cervical spine
(d) lateral view of the sternum

32. In making a posteroanterior radiograph of the chest, the shoulders are rolled forward primarily to:
(a) elevate the clavicles
(b) raise the diaphragm
(c) decrease the part-film distance
(d) move the scapulae laterally

33. That portion of the pelvis that articulates

with the femur to form the hip joint is called the:
(a) glenoid
(b) acromion
(c) malleolus
(d) acetabulum
(e) astragalus

34. That portion of a typical vertebra that is situated anteriorly is called the:
(a) pedicle
(b) body
(c) lamina
(d) transverse process
(e) spinous process

35. In positioning the skull for Stenver's position, the petrous portion of the temporal bone should be:
(a) 10 degrees to the film surface
(b) 45 degrees to the film surface
(c) 90 degrees to the film surface
(d) parallel to the film surface

36. In the examination of the paranasal sinuses, the erect position is *primarily* to:
(a) provide more comfort for the patient
(b) show fluid levels more accurately
(c) ease the pressure caused by sinusitis
(d) speed up the examination of the sinuses

37. The most satisfactory radiographic examination of a long bone suspected of being fractured should include:
(a) the joint proximal to the injury
(b) a similar bone for comparison
(c) the joint distal to the injury
(d) joints both proximal and distal to the injury

38. The five metacarpal bones are located in the:
(a) wrist
(b) ankle
(c) hand
(d) foot

39. The name of the "heel bone" is the:
(a) talus
(b) astragalus
(c) os navicularis
(d) os calcis

40. Which of the following combinations determines the thickness of the plane portrayed by body section radiography:
(a) length of tube travel and part-film distance
(b) target-film distance and length of tube travel
(c) part-film distance and speed of tube travel
(d) speed of tube travel and length of tube travel

41. Which one of the following diseases is *not* commonly seen in abdominal survey films:
(a) cholelithiasis
(b) nephrolithiasis
(c) bladder calculi
(d) polyps

42. Radiation kills most cells by:
(a) producing mutational changes in the chromosomes
(b) inhibiting cell division
(c) arresting DNA synthesis
(d) an interphase mechanism

43. The type of current supplied by the rectifier to the x-ray tube is best described as:
(a) alternating current
(b) constant current
(c) pulsating direct current
(d) direct current
(e) constant voltage

44. Poor vision particularly at night may be caused by:
(a) an excess of vitamin C
(b) a lack of vitamin B_1
(c) an excess of vitamin B_6
(d) a lack of vitamin D
(e) a lack of vitamin A

45. The term "ventral" is synonymous with:
(a) dorsal
(b) anterior
(c) proximal
(d) cranial
(e) caudal

46. The olecranon process of the ulna is situated_____to the styloid process of the radius.
(a) proximal
(b) anterior
(c) distal
(d) dorsal
(e) lateral

47. The five metacarpals of the hand articulate with the greater and lesser multangular bones, the capitate, and the:
(a) navicular
(b) lunate
(c) hamate
(d) triquetrum
(e) pisiform

48. The five metatarsals of the foot articulate with the first, second, and third cuneiforms and the:
(a) talus
(b) scaphoid
(c) navicular
(d) astragalus
(e) cuboid

49. The inverse square law does not hold true

for all types of radiation. For which of the following does it hold true:
- (a) electromagnetic
- (b) beta
- (c) alpha
- (d) neutrons
- (e) positrons

50. The severity of radiation sickness is:
- (a) dependent on the dose received and the type of tissue irradiated
- (b) unrelated to the dose received and dependent upon the energy of the incident radiation
- (c) dependent only on the type of tissue irradiated
- (d) dependent on the volume of tissue irradiated and independent of the dose received

51. The maximum permissible dose for radiation workers defined by the International Committee on Radiation Protection refers to the dose received from:
- (a) medical and occupational exposure
- (b) natural background radiation and occupational exposure
- (c) occupational exposure only
- (d) natural background, medical and occupational exposure

52. Which of the following instruments would be used to demonstrate the effect of kilovoltage on contrast:
- (a) spinning top
- (b) ballistics meter
- (c) oscilloscope
- (d) aluminum step wedge

53. When proper radiographic detail cannot be obtained because of excessive part-film distance, what change in technique may be used to improve the detail:
- (a) change the kvp
- (b) increase the time
- (c) change the mas
- (d) increase the focal-film distance

54. In radiography of the pubic symphysis, with the patient in the posteroanterior position, median plane in the midline of the table, and the central ray perpendicular to the film, the film and central ray should be centered at the level of the:
- (a) posterior-inferior iliac spine
- (b) anterior-superior iliac spine
- (c) greater trochanters
- (d) sacral promontory

55. The apophyseal articulations of the lumbar vertebrae are best visualized in:
- (a) lateral views
- (b) flexion views
- (c) oblique views
- (d) lateral bending views
- (e) extension views

56. In the posterior-anterior oblique projection for the sternoclavicular articulations, the affected side or the side being x-rayed is:
- (a) closest to the film
- (b) away from the film
- (c) closest to the tube
- (d) perpendicular to the ceiling
- (e) nearest the technician

57. In the bending positions of the wrist or with the wrist in ulnar or radial flexion or in the oblique semisupination and semipronation, the two carpal bones best demonstrated are:
- (a) navicular and talus
- (b) capitate and lunate
- (c) navicular and pisiform
- (d) cuneiform and calcis
- (e) scaphoid and cuboid

58. The greater the grid ratio, the greater the:
- (a) speed of exposure
- (b) radius of the grid
- (c) screening efficiency of the grid
- (d) focal-film distance required

59. When using a Bucky with a focused grid, if the lateral edges of the film lose density, it is an indication that the:
- (a) grid travels too fast
- (b) focal-film distance is too great
- (c) tube is not perpendicular to the grid
- (d) part-film distance is too great

60. A radiograph is made using a 16:1 ratio Bucky. The resulting film shows longitudinal streaks of uneven densities. These are probably caused by the:
- (a) central ray not being directed to the center of the table
- (b) Bucky moving unevenly during the exposure
- (c) Bucky stopping at some time during the exposure
- (d) film moving during the exposure

61. How much less is the exposure when no grid is used than when a 16:1 grid is used:
- (a) no change
- (b) one fourth as much
- (c) one sixth as much
- (d) one eighth as much

62. A plane made by cutting across the body from side to side at right angles to any sagittal plane is known as a:
- (a) midsagittal plane
- (b) coronal plane
- (c) transverse plane
- (d) median plane

63. Which of the following is a radiographic examination of the fluid-containing spaces of the brain:
    (a) carotid angiography
    (b) venography
    (c) pneumoencephalography
    (d) angiocardiography

64. A radiograph showing a complete lack of penumbra would be called:
    (a) sharp in detail
    (b) low in density
    (c) high in contrast
    (d) distorted

65. Underexposure of a radiograph may be caused by all of the following *except:*
    (a) kvp too low
    (b) mas too low
    (c) focal spot size too small
    (d) FFD too high

66. "The range between the minimum and maximum exposure that will produce a scale of translucent densities acceptable for diagnostic purposes"; this is a definition of:
    (a) contrast
    (b) wave amplitude
    (c) exposure latitude
    (d) absorption differential

67. The loop of the duodenum is shaped roughly like the letter "C" and encloses the head of the:
    (a) cecum
    (b) pylorus
    (c) spleen
    (d) pancreas
    (e) liver

68. In order to maintain a constant density, if the distance is tripled, the exposure (mas) must be:
    (a) multiplied by 3
    (b) multiplied by 9
    (c) divided by 3
    (d) divided by 9

69. Blood leaves the right ventricle of the heart and enters the lungs by way of the:
    (a) aorta
    (b) pulmonary artery
    (c) vena cava
    (d) carotid artery
    (e) pulmonary vein

70. The National Bureau of Standards Handbook No. 76 pertains to:
    (a) x-ray generation and usage
    (b) x-ray protection for the diagnostic range
    (c) x-ray protection up to 3 million volts
    (d) standards for taking films
    (e) standards for therapy

71. A three-phase x-ray generator operates on three single phase currents, each out of step by:
    (a) 110 degrees
    (b) 120 degrees
    (c) 12 degrees
    (d) 144 degrees

72. In a four-value tube, full-wave rectified circuit, during an exposure with a spinning top of $\frac{1}{10}$ second duration, there are how many dots noted if all systems work correctly:
    (a) 11
    (b) 14
    (c) 6
    (d) 12

73. A device used to increase the voltage of an alternating current by mutual induction between the primary and secondary coils is called:
    (a) a milliammeter
    (b) a step-down transformer
    (c) a step-up transformer
    (d) a step-up galvanometer

74. The set of screens in a rapid film changer should be:
    (a) cleaned only when the film jam-up takes place
    (b) cleaned periodically
    (c) never touched because of delicate balance
    (d) never exposed to white light

75. If a television monitor camera fails to function, the best approach would be:
    (a) to take off the housing and test it
    (b) to forget it and merely use the other systems available
    (c) call a serviceman who is qualified to repair it
    (d) call anyone in maintenance who has the proper tools

76. Image intensification tubes should not be exposed to raw radiation for any length of time because:
    (a) they will cause excessive radiation build-up
    (b) they will cause an overload of the fluoro tube
    (c) they will cause the image tube phosphors to form gas pockets
    (d) they will cause the image tube phosphors to change fluorescence

77. The optic lenses of any image intensification equipment should:
    (a) be cleaned with soap and water
    (b) be cleaned with ether or alcohol
    (c) not be cleaned at all
    (d) be wiped with a soft, lint-free cloth

78. A spinning top is used to find:

(a) detail sharpness
(b) radiographic quality
(c) time accuracy
(d) CVP accuracy

79. Which of these factors affects the quality of an x-ray beam:
(a) milliamperage
(b) length of exposure
(c) filter
(d) milliampere-seconds

80. The *chief* purpose of a filter of aluminum placed beneath the aperture of a radiographic tube is to:
(a) control the latitude of the radiographic image
(b) eliminate the light given off by the filament
(c) absorb some of the longer wavelengths
(d) filter out undesirable stem radiation

81. The four possible sets of technical factors listed below are to be used in routine radiography of a particular anatomic region. Select the set of factors that would most likely produce a radiograph with the *most magnification*, with all factors listed remaining the same:
(a) 25 mas, 1-mm. focal spot, 40-inch focal-film distance, 4-inch part-film distance
(b) 20 mas, 2-mm. focal spot, 36-inch focal-film distance, 4-inch part-film distance
(c) 25 mas, 2-mm. focal spot, 36-inch focal-film distance, 6-inch part-film distance
(d) 25 mas, 1-mm. focal spot, 40-inch focal-film distance, 6-inch part-film distance

82. Which of the following is easiest to penetrate radiographically:
(a) osteoporosis
(b) hydrocephalus
(c) osteopetrosis
(d) Paget's disease

83. All other factors being equal, the greatest radiographic density would be obtained by using an exposure of:
(a) 1/10 second and 100 ma
(b) 1/50 second and 300 ma
(c) 1/40 second and 500 ma
(d) 1/20 second and 200 ma

84. When making a radiographic exposure, the *primary* function of the mas is to:
(a) increase penetration
(b) regulate density
(c) regulate contrast
(d) increase contrast

85. The single mechanical factor that does the *most* to control radiographic detail is the:
(a) kilovoltage
(b) Potter-Bucky diaphragm

(c) object-film distance
(d) intensifying screen

86. In the development of exposed x-ray film, the action of the developer reduces silver salts to:
(a) grey metallic silver
(b) black metallic silver
(c) silver sulfide
(d) oxidized metallic silver

87. The *chief* cause of oxidation of the developer is:
(a) exposure to air
(b) high temperature
(c) impurities in the water
(d) exposure to unfiltered light

88. When sodium carbonate is used as a processing chemical for x-ray films, it serves as:
(a) a restrainer
(b) an accelerator
(c) a preservative
(d) a reducing agent

89. When sodium sulfite is used as an x-ray processing chemical, it is:
(a) a restrainer
(b) an accelerator
(c) a preservative
(d) a reducing agent

90. Three of the following are factors that determine the activity of the developer solution and one is not. Select the factor that does *not* determine the developer activity:
(a) agitation during development
(b) dilution of the developer
(c) development time
(d) chemicals in the developer

91. If a patient starts to vomit on the x-ray table, the technologist should:
(a) sit the patient up
(b) turn the patient's head to one side, avoiding aspiration
(c) bend the patient's legs
(d) turn the patient in prone position

92. The common duct is formed by the junction of:
(a) the cystic and one of the hepatic ducts
(b) the pancreatic and the cystic ducts
(c) the hepatic and the pancreatic ducts
(d) the cystic and the common hepatic ducts

93. T-tube cholangiography is done:
(a) before surgery of the gallbladder
(b) for diagnosis of stones in the pancreas
(c) after surgery of the gallbladder
(d) for diagnosis of nonobstructive jaundice

94. Industrial film is:
(a) used in body section radiography
(b) used in soft tissue studies of the neck

(c) not used in medical radiography

(d) used in mammography

95. In the intraoral projection for the submaxillary or sublingual glands, which of the following size films would you use:

(a) 8 × 10 nonscreen

(b) 5 × 7 nonscreen

(c) occlusal

(d) cine 70 mm.

(e) polaroid

96. An autotomogram during the erect filling phase of pneumoencephalogram is taken to demonstrate which of the following structures:

(a) fourth ventricle

(b) lateral ventricle

(c) corpus callosum

(d) anterior cerebral artery

97. A very small focal spot (0.3 mm.) is essential to obtain good:

(a) stereo views

(b) laminography

(c) magnification

(d) none of the above

98. Arthrography is done by injecting contrast media into:

(a) the bone

(b) the joint space

(c) the ligaments

(d) muscular fascia

99. Fractures of the facial bones are better demonstrated by:

(a) angiography

(b) osseous venography

(c) arthrography

(d) laminography

100. Viscosity refers to:

(a) contrast media

(b) any thick cohesive substance

(c) certain types of diseases

(d) a type of nerve operation

101. Jaundice is the result of damage to:

(a) white blood cells—leukolysis

(b) skin, from too much radiation

(c) bone, from repeated infections

(d) eyes, from direct sunlight

(e) the liver, as in hepatitis

102. Ballistic type mas meters are most useful in exposures where:

(a) x-ray tube current is small

(b) super-high kilovoltages are used

(c) exposure time is short

(d) exposure time is long

(e) x-ray tube current is large

103. Pathologic anatomy refers to:

(a) pathetic reactions

(b) condition of an organ or fluid produced by disease

(c) anatomy that is within normal limits

(d) embryonic or fetal disease

(e) normally functioning anatomy

104. Etiology is stated as the:

(a) study of ethnic groups of people

(b) science of logic

(c) science dealing with losses

(d) science of disease diagnosis

(e) study or theory of the causation of diseases

105. Diagnosis has to do with:

(a) distinguishing one disease from another

(b) a forecast of the probable result of a disease

(c) determining the order of a case

(d) the prospect for recovery

(e) determining the precise response the patient has to a treatment drug

106. Meatus means:

(a) one of the branches of the mandible

(b) the end of a long bone

(c) a long tubelike passage or canal

(d) the foramen magnum

107. The size and shape of the spleen, liver, and kidneys are best visualized in which of the following views of the abdomen:

(a) right anterior oblique

(b) anterior posterior supine

(c) lateral

(d) AP view with central ray horizontal

(e) decubitus

108. To demonstrate a fluid level in the chest or abdomen of a patient who is unable to be put in an erect position, which of the following positions might you use:

(a) supine

(b) Trendelenburg

(c) Fowler's

(d) lateral decubitus

(e) transthoracic

109. A cancer arising in bone is:

(a) sarcoma

(b) epithelial neoplasma

(c) basal cell carcinoma

(d) carcinoma of the fundus

(e) none of the above

110. The term LD 50/30 denotes the radiation dose required to kill:

(a) 50 percent of animals in thirty days

(b) 30 percent of animals in fifty days

(c) 50 percent of animals in fifty days

(d) 30 percent of animals in thirty days

111. When performing diagnostic radiology, the radiation absorbed in tissues is the result of what process:

(a) Compton interaction
(b) ionization
(c) photoelectric absorption
(d) excitation

112. Which of the following types of filtration is recommended for good mammography technique:
    (a) 1 mm. aluminum
    (b) 1 mm. copper
    (c) half-value layer
    (d) 1 mm. aluminum and 1 mm. beryllium
    (e) no filtration

113. A criterion for attaining satisfactory radiographic quality is:
    (a) minimum sharpness and true shape of the image
    (b) maximum sharpness and true shape of the image
    (c) densities are controlled by kvp primarily
    (d) contrast is controlled by milliampere seconds primarily

114. Cystoscopy would likely be involved in the examination called:
    (a) cholecystography
    (b) angiography
    (c) salpingography
    (d) retrograde urography

115. A drip infusion study is an examination of the:
    (a) fallopian tubes
    (b) bile ducts
    (c) salivary ducts
    (d) renal pelves

116. Which of the following is a radiographic examination of the uterus and tubes:
    (a) pelvimetry
    (b) cholangiography
    (c) hysterosalpingography
    (d) pneumoarthrography

117. Indicate which of the reasons below gives a valid excuse for withholding a meal prior to a radiographic examination:
    (a) gallbladder: the gallbladder may empty
    (b) excretory urogram: the kidneys may empty too fast
    (c) venogram: the veins will not fill properly
    (d) lumbar spine: the stomach will obscure the examination

118. Protective material in walls surrounding diagnostic x-ray machines is usually:
    (a) masonry
    (b) plaster
    (c) lead
    (d) glass
    (e) steel

119. When the filter in a diagnostic x-ray tube is increased, the effective wavelength of the useful beam is:
    (a) increased
    (b) decreased
    (c) not changed
    (d) changed directly, propositional to the filter
    (e) changed inversely, as the filter is changed

120. To comply with Handbook No. 76, the total filtration in the useful beam should be:
    (a) 1.0 mm. aluminum
    (b) 2.0 mm. aluminum
    (c) 3.0 mm. aluminum
    (d) not less than 2.5 mm. aluminum
    (e) 2.5 mm. aluminum

121. An increase in the kilovoltage across the x-ray tube results in:
    (a) radiation of shorter wavelength
    (b) radiation of longer wavelength
    (c) no alteration in wavelength
    (d) twice as many impulses per second
    (e) higher milliamperage

122. Three of the following are advantages of automatic processing of radiographic film and one is not. Select the one that is *not* an advantage:
    (a) it shortens the processing time
    (b) it diminishes the need for precise control of the temperature of solutions
    (c) it allows for better quality control
    (d) it increases the capacity of the radiology department or office because work flow is expedited

123. The base of x-ray film *may* be made of:
    (a) polyurethane
    (b) polyester
    (c) cellulose nitrate
    (d) silver bromide

124. Reticulation is the result of:
    (a) gross differences in temperatures between solutions
    (b) underdevelopment and overfixation
    (c) drying for short periods at high temperatures
    (d) negative charges built up inside of cassettes

125. The man who is called the "father of radioactivity" is:
    (a) Antoine Becquerel
    (b) Pierre Curie
    (c) Ernest Rutherford
    (d) Ed C. Jerman

126. Ethics is a discipline pertaining to:
    (a) good and bad behavior
    (b) intuition

(c) inductive reasoning

(d) English common law

127. In the following list of special examinations, which one does *not* belong in the series:
    (a) perirenal air insufflation
    (b) splenoportography
    (c) retrograde pyelography
    (d) nephrotomography

128. In which one of the following special examinations would a *higher* concentration of contrast medium most likely be used:
    (a) angiocardiography
    (b) intravenous urography
    (c) venography
    (d) cholangiography

129. The artificial contrast material used most frequently in studies of the vascular system is:
    (a) iodine
    (b) barium
    (c) air
    (d) carbon dioxide

130. Rapid filming methods are advantageous in which one of the following studies:
    (a) aortography
    (b) ventriculography
    (c) pneumoarthrography
    (d) retroperitoneal air studies

131. In the following list of special examinations, which one does *not* belong in the series:
    (a) pneumoencephalography
    (b) ventriculography
    (c) cerebral angiography
    (d) nephrotomography

132. The *primary* purpose of a pelvimetry examination is to determine the measurements of the:
    (a) fetus and placenta
    (b) pelvis
    (c) fetal head
    (d) fetal age

133. Radiation doses to the occupational personnel are measured in units of:
    (a) rem
    (b) rep
    (c) rad
    (d) roentgen
    (e) RBE

134. Pathology is the:
    (a) science dealing with the cause and course of the disease
    (b) science dealing with the nature of orderly function
    (c) program of treatment for a specific disease
    (d) treatment of disease with new drugs
    (e) science dealing with pathos of logic

135. Which of the following are visualized best in the Valdini position when the infraorbital-meatal line forms a 50-degree angle with the film:
    (a) external auditory canal and foramen ovale
    (b) sella turcica and dorsum sella
    (c) labyrinths and internal auditory canals
    (d) foramina spinosum and magnum
    (e) cochlea and auditory ossicles

136. Which of the following should be used to explain to a patient that he does not own his x-ray films:
    (a) he would have no use for them
    (b) he wouldn't know how to interpret them
    (c) the hospital owns them
    (d) they are a part of his permanent records at the hospital

137. Aseptic or sterile technique must be used:
    (a) for all procedures
    (b) whenever the skin is broken or penetrated
    (c) when known pathogenic organisms are present
    (d) whenever the patient is unable to swallow

138. When radiographing patients with infectious diseases, it is not necessary to:
    (a) wash the hands
    (b) wear a gown and mask
    (c) disinfect the x-ray equipment
    (d) avoid touching the patient

139. The use of motion in a radiograph can be utilized to the best advantage in the following:
    (a) PA view of ankle
    (b) oblique view of sternum
    (c) oblique view of ribs
    (d) lateral view of sacrum
    (e) AP view of cervical spine (levels 3 to 7)

140. Check the answer that is *not* correct. The sharpness of detail in a radiograph is primarily dependent upon:
    (a) the mass
    (b) the size of the focal spot
    (c) the target-film distance
    (d) immobilization
    (e) the object-film distance

141. The compounds used in fluoroscopic screens as a fluorescent agent are:
    (a) calcium carbonate
    (b) zinc oxide
    (c) zinc sulfide
    (d) zinc cadmium sulfide
    (e) silver sulfide

142. All but one of the following is importantly

related to the viscosity of a contrast medium.
Identify the exception:
(a) its content of iodine per molecule
(b) its ability to outline mucosal patterns
(c) the speed with which it can be injected
(d) the amount of leakage in the uterotubo-gram
(e) its ability to outline small bronchi and not alveoli

143. In manual processing procedures, to obtain the maximum density and contrast the generally accepted time and temperature for the development of screen-type film is:
(a) three minutes at 68°
(b) three minutes at 80°
(c) five minutes at 65°
(d) five minutes at 68°

144. Chemical processing stains on intensifying screens will cause —— on the finished radiograph.
(a) increased base fog
(b) light spots
(c) dark spots
(d) decreased base fog

145. Goiters are found in the:
(a) adrenal gland
(b) parotid gland
(c) thyroid gland
(d) shoulder muscles
(e) gluteal muscles

146. The chief purpose of the sodium thiosulfate in the fixing solution is to:
(a) harden the film emulsion
(b) remove the undeveloped silver salts
(c) stop the action of the developer
(d) remove the exposed silver

147. The reduction of silver salts to metallic silver during development of the latent image is accomplished by:
(a) sodium thiosulfate and sodium carbonate
(b) the action of light at low levels
(c) potassium bromide and sodium sulfite
(d) metol and hydroquinone

148. During a 100 ma exposure with full-wave rectified equipment, an accurate milliammeter indicates only 50 ma. It is possible that:
(a) the high-tension transformer has developed a short-circuit
(b) a valve tube is not functioning properly
(c) the timer is set improperly
(d) one of the fuses is burned out

149. Esophageal varices result from:
(a) strong allergic reactions to food
(b) cirrhosis of the liver
(c) pelvic vein obstruction

(d) injured leg
(e) collateral circulation associated with a brain lesion

150. Disease of the pancreas directly affects production of:
(a) digestive enzymes
(b) urine
(c) cerebrospinal fluid
(d) hair growth
(e) thyroid hormone

151. One of the main groups of pathogenic bacteria is:
(a) calculus
(b) malaria
(c) magnus
(d) coccus
(e) annulus

152. An important cause of lung abscess is:
(a) bronchiectasis
(b) intussusception
(c) biliary tract stasis
(d) nephrolithiasis
(e) cold air

153. A compound fracture is:
(a) a fracture that has two broken parts
(b) any fracture in many pieces
(c) any fracture that has broken through the skin
(d) only those fractures in many pieces that have broken through the skin

154. A foreign particle disease of the lung, pneumoconiosis, is:
(a) pneumococcus
(b) streptococcus
(c) filariasis
(d) lung flukes
(e) silicosis

155. Carbon dioxide may be preferred to air as a retroperitoneal contrast medium because:
(a) it is cleaner
(b) it is absorbed more quickly
(c) it is more opaque
(d) it is less opaque
(e) it is cheaper than oxygen

156. The use of ginger ale or other soft drinks as a contrast medium for double-contrast examination of the stomach depends on:
(a) the viscosity
(b) the sugar content
(c) the specific gravity
(d) the carbonation
(e) the ability to suspend the barium particles because of the stickiness of these drinks

157. If an x-ray tube is gassy, it will *usually* be noted that:

(a) no reading is obtained on the primary voltmeter
(b) the tube filament does not light up
(c) there are irregular fluctuations in the milliamperage
(d) the milliammeter does not register
(e) the valve tubes do not light up

158. Roentgen published his findings under the title of:
(a) "A New Kind of Ray"
(b) "How to Take a Good Radiograph"
(c) "The Story of X-Rays"
(d) "X-Rays and Dr. Roentgen"

159. The bronchogram is a radiographic examination of the:
(a) trachea
(b) larynx
(c) pharynx
(d) lung
(e) bronchi and their branches

160. Geriatrics is:
(a) the study of genes
(b) the study of elderly people
(c) the study of disease
(d) the study of children

161. A gene is:
(a) a biologic unit of heredity
(b) one of the twenty-four factors that tell what a human will look like
(c) an article of clothing
(d) the covering of all ameboid cells

162. To produce and discover the first known x-rays, Mr. Roentgen used a partially evacuated tube known as:
(a) Faraday tube
(b) Coolidge tube
(c) Langmuir tube
(d) Crookes-Hittorf tube

163. The fourth ventricle is located in the:
(a) posterior fossa
(b) middle fossa
(c) anterior fossa
(d) sella turcica

164. Erythema is:
(a) the evacuation of capillaries
(b) any congestion of capillaries causing an abnormal redness of skin
(c) shedding or peeling of dry skin
(d) skin with multiple cracks and pustules

165. One may enlist the aid of the patient more readily by:
(a) showing distaste at unpleasant or disturbing situations
(b) explaining procedure to him
(c) not including him in conversation

166. The three main groups of disease processes are:

(a) jaundice, glycosuria, and high white blood count
(b) inflammation, degeneration, and tumification
(c) symptoms of the eyes, skin, and nervous system
(d) the digestive system, nervous system, and endocrine system

167. Bone infection is called:
(a) osteomyelitis
(b) myelogenesis
(c) multiple myeloma
(d) osteology
(e) phrenology

168. Scurvy is caused by a:
(a) vitamin C excess
(b) vitamin deficiency
(c) hormone excess
(d) hormone deficiency
(e) genetic malformation

169. Inflammation of the gallbladder is:
(a) meningitis
(b) peritonitis
(c) coenzymitis
(d) cholecystitis
(e) calculitis

170. Currently used arteriography contrast agents *all* contain:
(a) sodium
(b) meglamine (methyl glucamine)
(c) iodine
(d) benzene

171. On November 8, 1895, W. C. Roentgen discovered x-rays at:
(a) the University of Zurich
(b) the Academy of Sciences in Paris
(c) the University of Wurtzburg
(d) Oxford University

172. A patient's chest measures 23 cm. in the anteroposterior diameter. Laminograms are to be made in the anteroposterior position of a questionable lesion 3 cm. posterior to the anterior chest wall. The fulcrum should be set at:
(a) 3 cm. from the tabletop
(b) 3 cm. above the midplane of the chest
(c) 20 cm. from the tabletop
(d) 23 cm. from the tabletop

173. Which of the following is not part of the kidney anatomy:
(a) pelvis
(b) calyx
(c) utricle
(d) medulla
(e) infundibulum

174. Exostosis, osteoma, and osteoporosis are:

(a) abnormal conditions of reproductive systems
(b) abnormal conditions of bones
(c) normal conditions of bones
(d) congenital anomalies

175. Information relating to a patient's condition or prognosis:
    (a) may be freely discussed with close relatives
    (b) must always remain confidential
    (c) should always be in open discussion since "a well-known fact is not a secret fact"
    (d) should be discussed only on a co-worker–interdepartmental basis

176. One of the following is not a classification of joints:
    (a) synarthrosis
    (b) dolychocephalic
    (c) amphiarthrotic
    (d) diarthrotic

177. A prefix:
    (a) comes before a word to alter the meaning
    (b) comes before a word to modify and enhance the word
    (c) comes after words to alter their meaning
    (d) is the same thing as a stem or root word

178. Epi, endo, peri, and ortho are:
    (a) terms used in the same manner as root words
    (b) terms describing opposites
    (c) suffixes
    (d) prefixes

179. The portal vein is formed by the joining of which of the following:
    (a) the left renal and superior mesenteric veins
    (b) the splenic and left renal veins
    (c) the superior and inferior mesenteric veins
    (d) the splenic and superior mesenteric veins
    (e) the splenic and hepatic veins

180. The most useful procedure in the evaluation of liver cirrhosis is:
    (a) superior mesenteric arteriogram
    (b) lumbar aortogram
    (c) percutaneous cholangiogram
    (d) splenoportogram
    (e) renal arteriogram

181. CO_2 is used for retroperitoneal insufflation because:
    (a) it gives better density than air
    (b) it is readily dissolved in blood
    (c) patients laugh louder than when nitrous oxide is used

(d) it is excreted by the kidney
(e) it demonstrates renal vasculature

182. Which of the following should be used to answer a patient's inquiry as to his x-ray findings:
    (a) give him a brief summary of what has been said about his films
    (b) explain his x-ray findings in detail, including reading him the written report
    (c) explain to him that everyone is very busy and he'll get his report as soon as possible
    (d) explain that you cannot give him a report but that you will mention his request to his doctor

183. Branches of the aortic arch include all of the following except:
    (a) innominate artery
    (b) left subclavian artery
    (c) right common carotid artery
    (d) left common carotid artery

184. Pelvic pneumography is a technique whereby the pelvic structures are outlined by a negative contrast agent such as one of the following:
    (a) room air
    (b) oxygen
    (c) nitrous ovide
    (d) compressed air
    (e) water density fluid

185. Diabetes makes a patient more susceptible to:
    (a) tumors
    (b) oxygen
    (c) infections
    (d) halogens
    (e) ozone

186. Pneumonia may be caused by:
    (a) viruses
    (b) cold air
    (c) increased respiratory rate
    (d) increased skin permeability
    (e) warm respiratory gases

187. A cholangiogram is used to visualize the:
    (a) bile ducts
    (b) parotid ducts
    (c) salivary ducts
    (d) lymph ducts

188. The fetal skeleton is first evident by x-ray at:
    (a) six weeks
    (b) fifteen to sixteen weeks
    (c) twenty-seven to twenty-eight weeks
    (d) thirty-six weeks
    (e) forty weeks

189. Secondary radiation is produced whenever:
    (a) primary radiation is incident on material bodies

(b) the frequency of x-rays increases

(c) the anode potential of the x-ray tube decreases to zero

(d) the anode potential of the x-ray tube reaches its peak value

(e) x-rays pass through a magnetic field

190. Disease in the pituitary gland is a direct cause of:
    (a) gigantism
    (b) lung collapse
    (c) increased phlegm
    (d) pneumoconiosis
    (e) hay fever

191. A form of leukemia is called:
    (a) autogenous
    (b) paralytic
    (c) lymphatic
    (d) homogenous
    (e) emphatic

192. Calcification in fibroids, often seen on a plain film of the abdomen, is in the:
    (a) uterus
    (b) annulus
    (c) spine
    (d) ureter
    (e) psoas shadows

193. Chronic mastitis is an inflammatory change of the:
    (a) foot
    (b) mastoid
    (c) breast
    (d) elbow
    (e) hands

194. High blood pressure, hypertension, follows:
    (a) a partial block of a renal artery
    (b) a rapid hemorrhage
    (c) the release of a substance by a diseased tophus
    (d) a sudden lung collapse
    (e) a severe state of shock

195. A low output of hormone by the thyroid gland causes:

    (a) hypoparathyroidism
    (b) cretinism
    (c) Addison's disease
    (d) mixed areola
    (e) a desire for salt

196. The foramina ovale, spinosum, lacerum, jugulare, and magnum are best seen in which of the following views of the skull:
    (a) fronto-occipital view
    (b) submentovertical view
    (c) Caldwell's view
    (d) Towne's view
    (e) intraoral view

197. The diaphysis is:
    (a) the primary center of ossification
    (b) the end or extremity of a long bone
    (c) the secondary center of ossification
    (d) a general term used to describe the bones of a fetus

198. Translucent means:
    (a) born color-blind
    (b) a condition of the lungs
    (c) that light can penetrate
    (d) that light cannot penetrate

199. Body section radiography employs the principle of:
    (a) motion, distortion, and unsharpness during exposure
    (b) an optical illusion
    (c) a tridimensional image
    (d) a tridimensional image and an optional illustration

200. The proximal portion of the stomach is referred to as the:
    (a) fundus
    (b) pylorus
    (c) antrum
    (d) lesser curvature
    (e) greater curvature

SIMULATED REGISTRY EXAMINATION II ANSWER SHEET

1.	b	26.	d	51.	c	76.	c	101.	e	126.	a	151.	d	176.	b
2.	b	27.	b	52.	d	77.	d	102.	c	127.	b	152.	a	177.	b
3.	d	28.	b	53.	d	78.	c	103.	b	128.	a	153.	c	178.	d
4.	b	29.	b	54.	c	79.	c	104.	e	129.	a	154.	e	179.	d
5.	d	30.	c	55.	c	80.	c	105.	a	130.	a	155.	b	180.	d
6.	b	31.	c	56.	a	81.	c	106.	c	131.	d	156.	d	181.	b
7.	a	32.	d	57.	c	82.	a	107.	b	132.	b	157.	c	182.	d
8.	d	33.	d	58.	c	83.	c	108.	d	133.	a	158.	a	183.	c
9.	a	34.	b	59.	b	84.	b	109.	a	134.	a	159.	e	184.	c
10.	a	35.	d	60.	a	85.	c	110.	a	135.	b	160.	b	185.	c
11.	d	36.	b	61.	c	86.	b	111.	c	136.	d	161.	a	186.	a
12.	a	37.	d	62.	c	87.	a	112.	e	137.	b	162.	d	187.	a
13.	d	38.	c	63.	c	88.	b	113.	b	138.	d	163.	a	188.	b
14.	b	39.	d	64.	a	89.	c	114.	d	139.	b	164.	b	189.	a
15.	e	40.	b	65.	c	90.	c	115.	d	140.	a	165.	b	190.	a
16.	b	41.	d	66.	c	91.	b	116.	c	141.	d	166.	b	191.	c
17.	a	42.	b	67.	d	92.	d	117.	a	142.	a	167.	a	192.	a
18.	a	43.	c	68.	b	93.	c	118.	c	143.	d	168.	b	193.	c
19.	d	44.	e	69.	b	94.	d	119.	b	144.	b	169.	d	194.	a
20.	c	45.	b	70.	c	95.	c	120.	d	145.	c	170.	c	195.	b
21.	c	46.	a	71.	b	96.	a	121.	a	146.	b	171.	c	196.	b
22.	c	47.	c	72.	d	97.	c	122.	b	147.	d	172.	c	197.	a
23.	b	48.	e	73.	c	98.	b	123.	b	148.	b	173.	e	198.	c
24.	c	49.	a	74.	b	99.	d	124.	a	149.	b	174.	b	199.	a
25.	a	50.	a	75.	c	100.	b	125.	a	150.	a	175.	b	200.	a

INDEX

219